# THE
# GARDEN
## APOTHECARY

# THE
# GARDEN
# APOTHECARY

*Homemade remedies*
*for everyday ailments*

## REECE CARTER

NON
FICTION
HQ

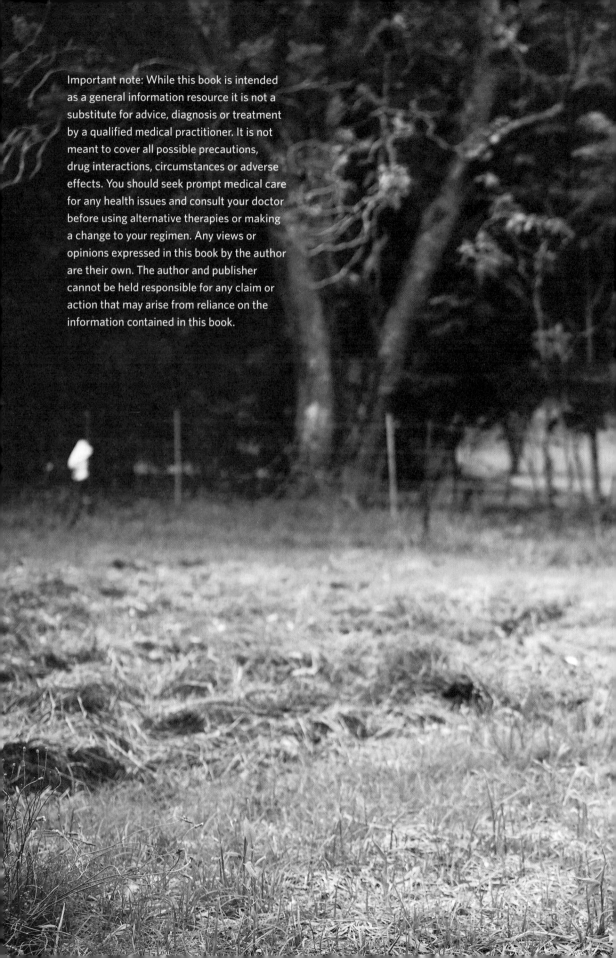

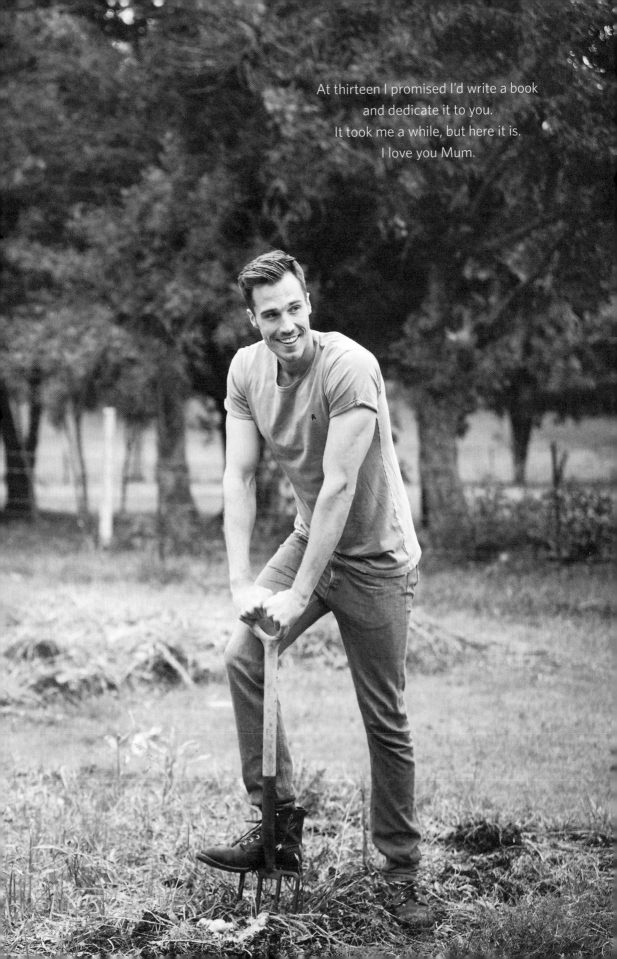

At thirteen I promised I'd write a book
and dedicate it to you.
It took me a while, but here it is.
I love you Mum.

# CONTENTS

## INTRODUCING HERBAL MEDICINE

Why use natural remedies?
11

Getting started
18

Growing a garden apothecary
28

Stocking the pantry
47

## THE REMEDIES

Basic techniques
54

Natural beauty: Recipes for skin and hair health
66

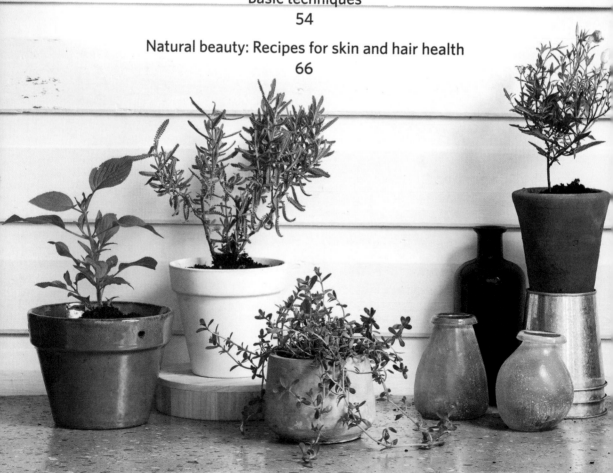

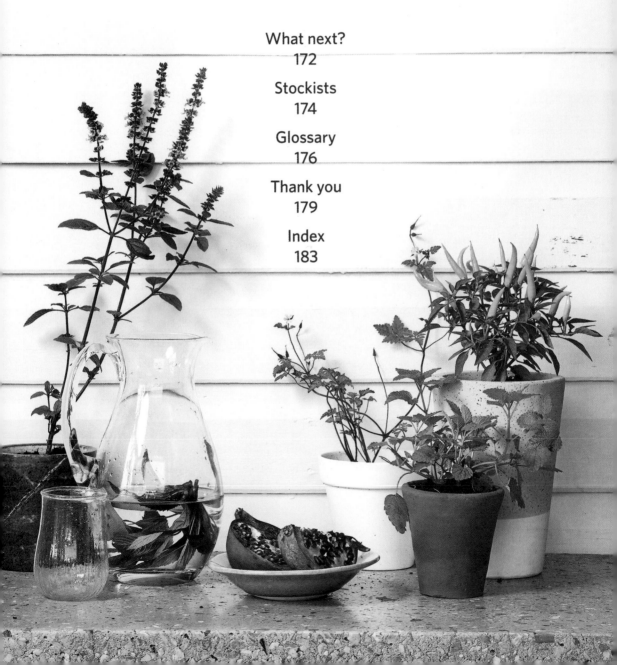

Forever young: Remedies to boost energy, mood and libido
92

Daily rhythm: A herbal approach to stress and sleep management
112

Gut instinct: Your guide to bloating, indigestion and other tummy troubles
130

Flu fighters: Immune system tonics for colds, flus and allergies
148

What next?
172

Stockists
174

Glossary
176

Thank you
179

Index
183

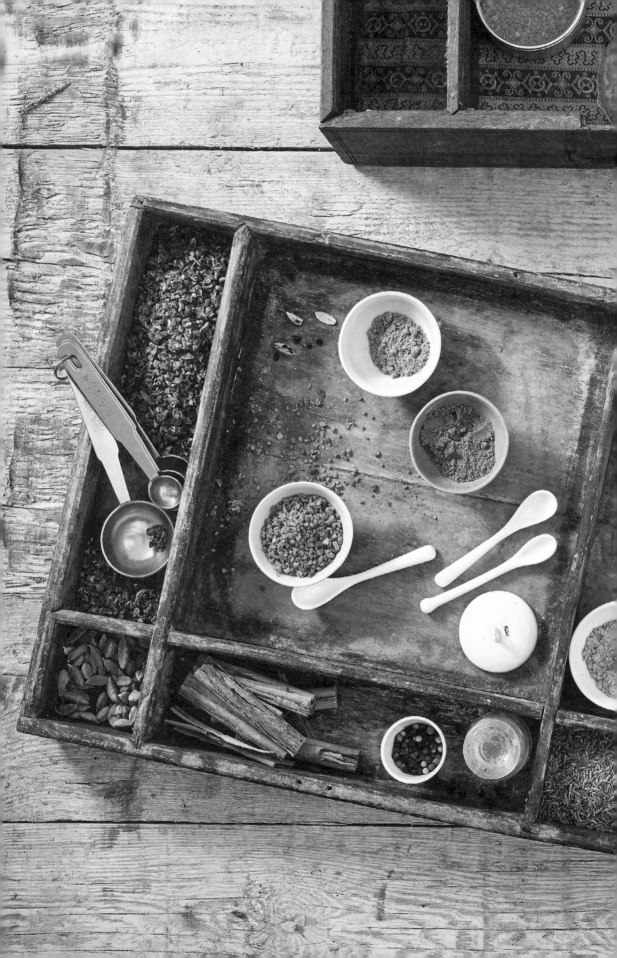

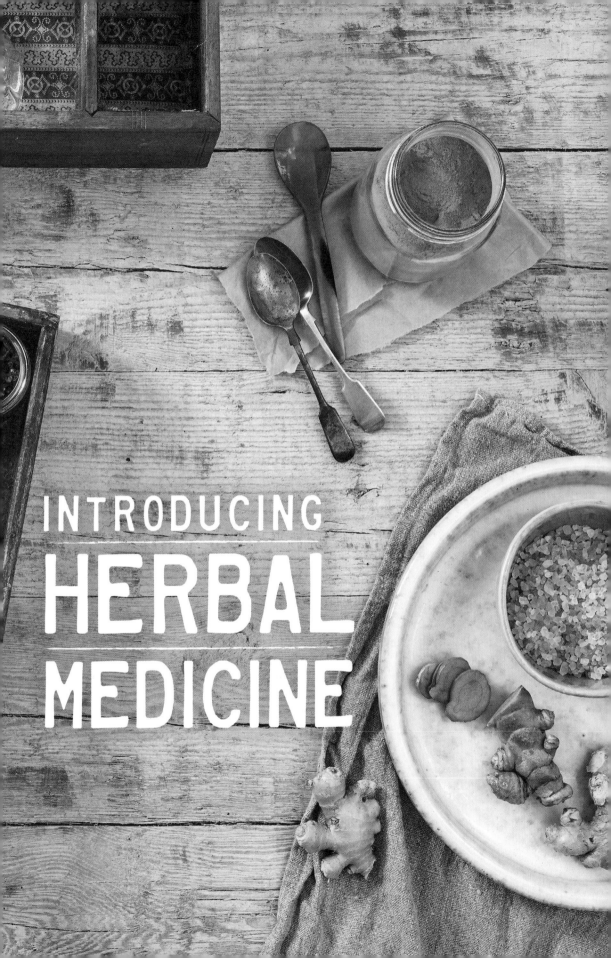

# INTRODUCING
# HERBAL
# MEDICINE

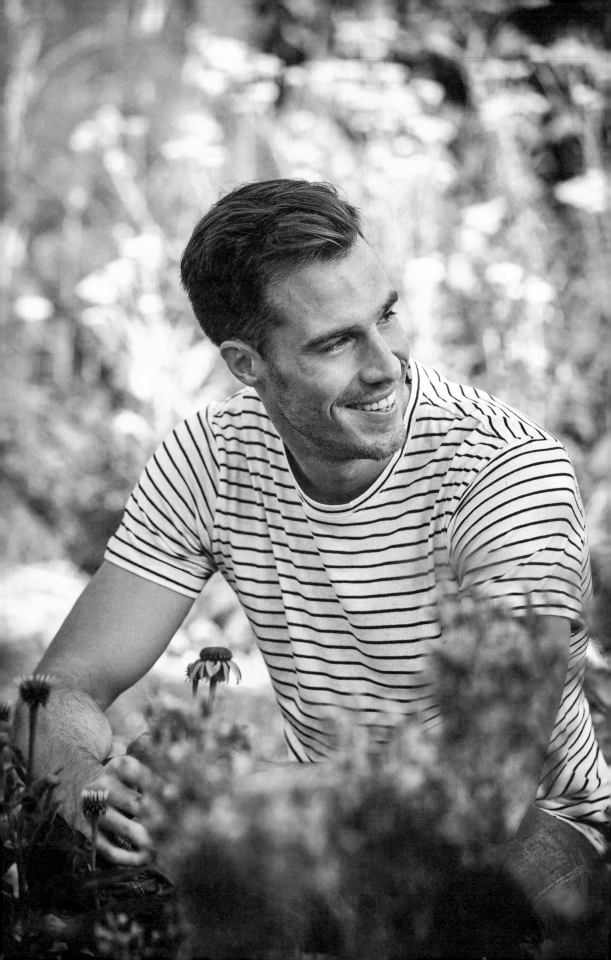

# WHY USE NATURAL REMEDIES?

*A gentle way to manage day-to-day ailments*

**HOME REMEDIES HAVE** grown to be important to me because they offer a very gentle way to manage day-to-day ailments. To me, the philosophy that underpins herbal medicine just makes good sense: treat the root cause and do so as gently as possible. Rather than suppressing the body's natural processes, herbal medicine works alongside them to correct imbalances 'from the ground up', and not just cover up the symptoms. I realised just *how* important to me they had become when my friends came up with the nickname 'Herb nerd'. They would come over to my house, go to grab a snack and instead be confronted with a confusing pantry packed with amber bottles and ointment-filled jars. Even getting in and out of the house was tricky, with my herb garden taking over the front yard like some inner-city jungle. That's what you get for being a naturopath with a passion for all things green. For me, this journey began as a green-thumbed kid, running around Pop's incredible vegetable garden enjoying a mouthful of gooseberries. I'd try to replicate it as a small veggie patch of my own back on our farm—with results that never quite matched Pop's—and make a total mess of the kitchen. I'm happy to say that both habits are alive and well today.

Fast forward to my teens and, longing to fill out my wiry frame, I discovered the gym. This interest in fitness naturally grew to include nutrition too, and by my twenties I had toppled headfirst into the rabbit hole that is food as medicine and natural wellness. My idea of a good time was researching how the food we ate impacted our health. It didn't take long before I was also devouring information about traditional remedies and ancient medicines. Driven to know more—and realising that the conflicting views of Google might not be entirely reliable—I decided to get a more formal education on the topic. I moved to Melbourne and enrolled in a degree in Health Science. It was there that my passion for herbal medicine was really ignited.

My herb garden grew to include not only parsley and basil, but also a whole host of herbs that could be used to treat specific ailments, like echinacea for immunity or valerian to help bring on sleep. Trips to the hardware store became a weekly event, allowing me to buy more timber to build planter boxes for my brahmi—a great memory tonic, if you were wondering (see page 35)—and recycled pots to fill with calendula, my favourite herb for skin health.

And while my training is particularly focused on Western European herbalism, the same philosophies are echoed in all of the great natural medicine traditions: treat the cause, and do so gently. Throughout my journey, I picked up little nuggets of wisdom from Chinese medicine and Ayurveda—an ancient form of medicine used largely in India and Sri Lanka—which helped shape my approach to home-grown healthcare.

# WHY *MAKE* YOUR OWN REMEDIES?

Before pharmacists, there were apothecaries. These people largely concerned themselves with turning plant life into medicines which they would sell from their stores; they were the healers of the time.

And there was something ever-so-slightly magical about the way they worked, with their amber glass jars and age-old methods. It's a practice jam-packed with tradition. But as the human race has evolved, so too has our understanding of how these herbs work. Scientific discovery has enriched the practice of herbalism. For me, understanding the *science* of herbs is as important as knowing about their traditional uses. Knowing the names and actions of the individual compounds that lend a plant its medicinal actions helps highlight new ways to use that plant, and so traditional medicines fuse with current scientific understanding to carve out a place for herbs in contemporary healthcare.

I suppose I shouldn't be surprised, then, that this is the field I've ended up working in. When asked as a child what I wanted to be when I grew up, my answer was invariably either a scientist—I imagined all scientists to be Einstein-looking geniuses brewing secret concoctions and making test tubes explode—or a magician. Somehow, I've landed between the two.

Even in the world of pharmaceuticals, there are traces of herbalism: it is estimated that around 70 per cent of all drugs have their roots, once upon a time, in herbal medicine. It was when apothecaries began to dabble in this wholesale production of drugs from plants that the pharmaceutical industry was born. Eventually, the plants themselves were no longer needed and the same drugs could be synthesised in laboratories. Non plant-based medications came along not long after, and pretty soon herbal medicine found itself labelled archaic and ineffective. People began to mistrust natural therapies—until their recent resurgence in popularity, that is.

> Scientific discovery has enriched the practice of herbalism.

Today, the natural supplement industry is big business. People are once again embracing herbal healthcare, this time alongside modern medicine. But whereas now we think of herbal medicine as products to purchase, it once required a set of skills.

People didn't go out and buy a supplement; they got hands-on in the brewing of a remedy. Somebody in the household (usually Mum) would know which humble occupants of the spice rack could cure a cold, which foods would give glowing skin and which herbs could help a troubled sleeper. These skills are largely gone—apart from a few pockets of nerdy enthusiasts like myself—but what if they weren't? What if you knew you had a planter box full of sleep on your windowsill, and a jar full of pain-relief sitting in your pantry?

We're all about detoxing these days—detoxing our homes, detoxing our bodies—so how about detoxing the medicine cabinet? This is not to say there isn't a time and place for pharmaceuticals, because of course there is. Modern medical treatments save lives, there is no doubt about that, and this book isn't intended as a replacement for prescribed medication or proper medical care. Home remedies are not meant to take the place of your existing medications, but rather to complement them and assist in the management of your day-to-day wellness, alongside healthy diet and exercise. It's important to follow your doctor's orders, prioritise your prescribed medications, and if in doubt always consult a health professional before making any changes—even natural ones!

But for many of those daily health woes and minor annoyances, a gentle, organic remedy could be the answer. We have all,

> Whereas now we think of herbal medicine as products to purchase, it once required a set of skills.

at some stage, suffered a sleepless night or become frustrated at sniffles that just won't stop. These are the situations where knowing your passionflower from your elderflower becomes invaluable. And if you don't know the difference yet, you will soon.

For many of these chronic complaints, you may actually find that natural medicine has an answer when your pharmacy falls short. Herbs really shine because they work in harmony with your body's own processes, rather than interrupting them. They nourish and support the body's homeostatic—that means 'balancing'—processes, and keep your body working at its best. When it comes to issues like stress, insomnia and digestion in particular, giving the body the help it needs to heal itself is often the best tactic, and that's exactly what natural medicine does.

Here in Australia, we're starting to see a real shift towards a more holistic form of healthcare. People are becoming aware of the fact that for long-term wellness, we need to consider preventative health strategies.

We have all, at some stage, suffered a sleepless night or become frustrated at sniffles that just won't stop. These are the situations where knowing your passionflower from your elderflower becomes invaluable.

about how herbs were used traditionally and what we know about them today. You'll discover how to combine them to maximise their effects, what doses to use them in and—perhaps most importantly—how to effectively extract all their medicinal goodness and turn them into *effective* remedies. I will give you advice on growing your plants and keeping them healthy, guidance on which herbs to use for different conditions and tips on how herbs can be integrated into your lifestyle as preventative health measures. You'll also find clear and simple recipes that show you how to make your own remedies cheaply at home.

*The Garden Apothecary* is designed to empower and excite you to take charge of your health. It's a start-to-finish guide that helps you take care of yourself and your family naturally. It's your almanac for making old medicines new again.

These are largely nutritional considerations, and so the food-as-medicine movement is booming. Whether you're a paleo devotee, vegan, a raw foodie or like me just an advocate for eating real food, one thing is clear: healthy eating is back, and in a big way. People are learning to cook wholefoods again, paying attention to what they are putting in their bodies, and taking control of their health through a nourishing diet.

The next big thing in this wellness revolution then—at least in my humble herb-nerd opinion—is the return of condition-specific treatments that can be plucked from your garden or whipped up in your kitchen. Simply put, it's time to relearn the art and the science of herbal medicine, and discover how to relieve many common ailments with the exact same things that you put on your plate.

And that's exactly what we're going to do. In *The Garden Apothecary* you'll learn

It's time to relearn the art and the science of herbal medicine, and discover how to relieve many common ailments with the same things that you put on your plate.

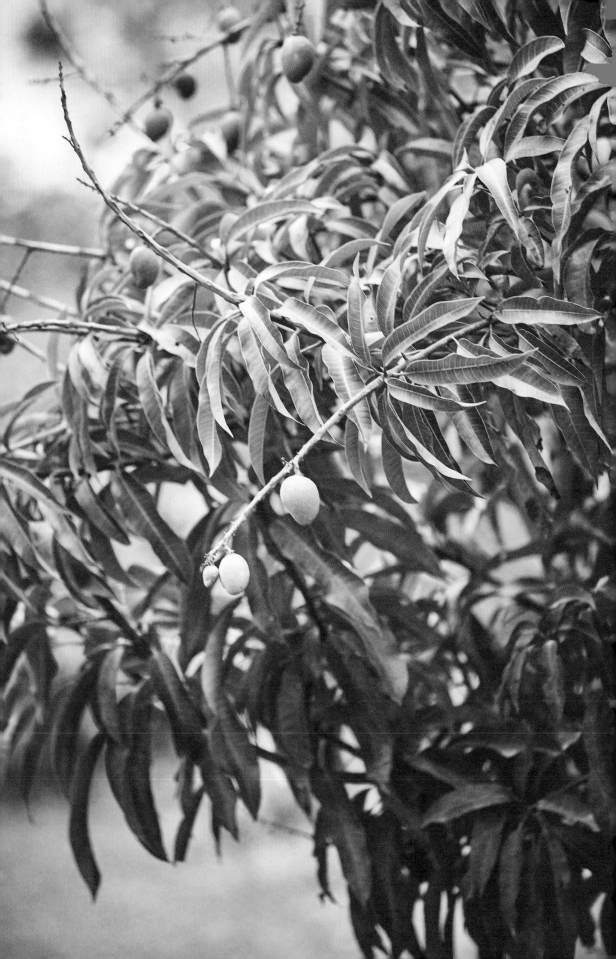

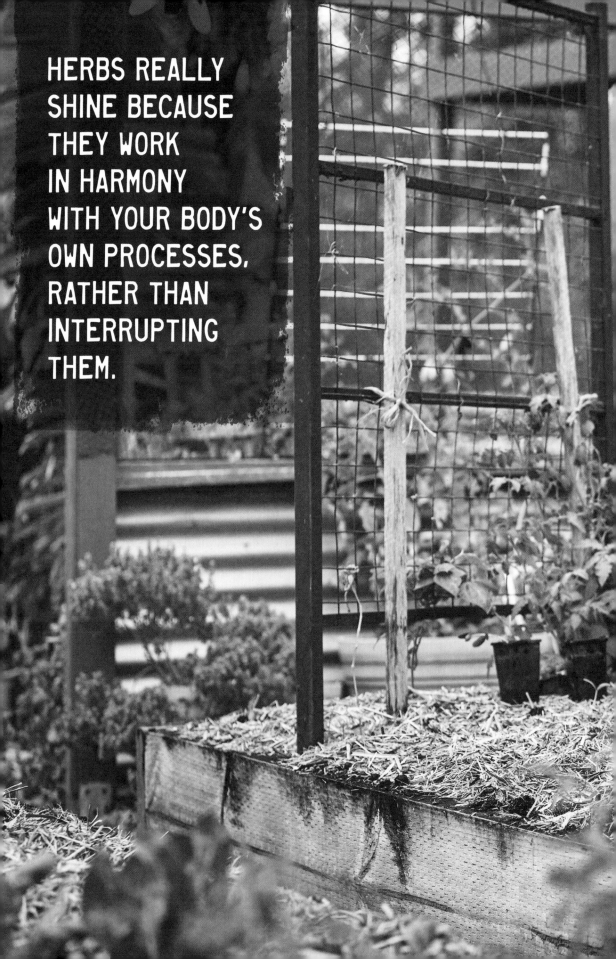

HERBS REALLY SHINE BECAUSE THEY WORK IN HARMONY WITH YOUR BODY'S OWN PROCESSES, RATHER THAN INTERRUPTING THEM.

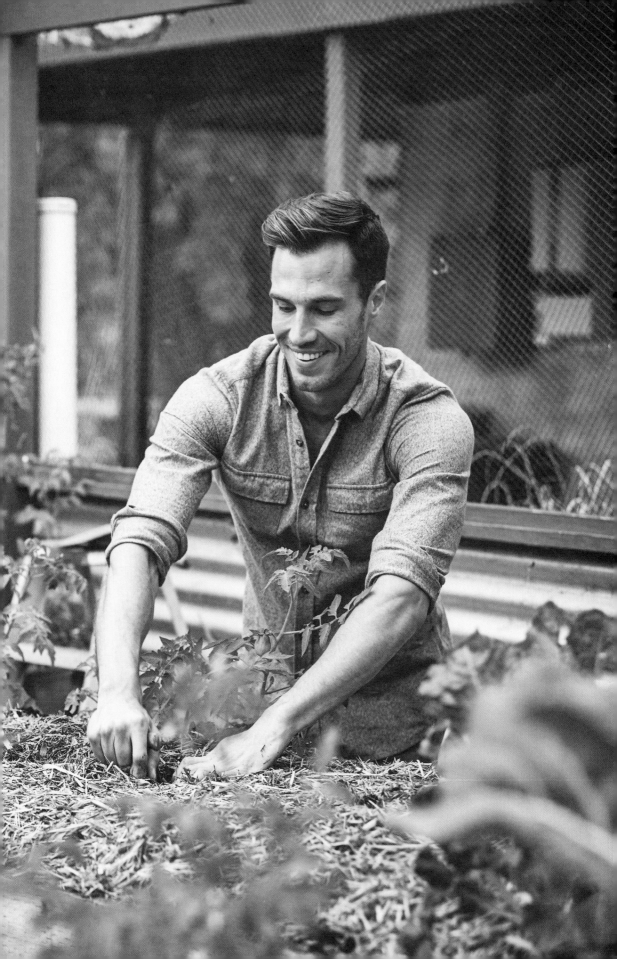

# GETTING STARTED

*Everything a budding herbalist needs to know.*

**IT MAY SEEM** a daunting and strange new task to become your own medicine-maker, but you don't need to have a flourishing garden or a towering stockpile of tinctures. Believe it or not, you've probably got enough in your kitchen pantry to get started right now. Check those little glass jars of powdered spices, the ones tucked away in the back of your pantry. Got cloves? Then you hold in your hands one of nature's best anaesthetics for toothache and painful ulcers. See that cinnamon? It's the perfect remedy to tame a sweet tooth. And that bright yellow powder? That's turmeric, the king of herbal anti-inflammatories.

The other good news is that the methods are pretty easy and you don't have to be a chef or a botanist to turn plants into medicine. Sometimes, it's as simple as grabbing a bunch of greenery from the garden and chewing on it. I can't tell you how grateful I've been for a handful of raw parsley after overindulging on garlic at dinner—in hindsight, my companions were probably pretty grateful for it too!

There are a few classic methods that herbalists use to make remedies and they all involve extracting and concentrating the active compounds from raw herbs or spices in water, in oil or in vodka. The extraction you choose to make will depend on the herb itself and the intended finished product. From there, once you've got the extract you need, it can be turned into more complex remedies. Ultimately, it will be the purpose

> The methods are pretty easy and you don't have to be a chef or a botanist to turn plants into medicine.

of the medicine that will determine which one you make. I've outlined the major forms of herbal medicine below, as well as when to use them.

# TINCTURES

Tinctures, or fluid extracts, are the bread-and-butter of the modern herbalist. They are a mix of alcohol and water that draw out and dissolve the bits of the herbs that you want to use. With that said, it makes sense that you'd need a source of ethanol (pure alcohol) and water, and so spirits are the ideal choice for home remedies. Vodka, being a colourless alcohol with no obvious taste, is my pick of the bunch. If you can't take alcohol or are making remedies for children, a mixture of food-grade vegetable glycerine and water can be used instead. We call this a *glycetract*. These also work when you need to make a thicker remedy, for example, when you're making something to coat a sore throat.

# INFUSED OILS

Infused oils are basically tinctures made with oil instead of alcohol or glycerine. They are used externally and make amazing skin, hair and nail treatments. Oils can be loaded with skin-soothing and wound-healing ingredients and applied directly to your skin, or poured into your bath. Just take your base oil and make it like you would a tincture. The one downside? They tend to leave the skin oily, and don't absorb as well as creams or lotions.

# CREAMS AND LOTIONS

Both creams and lotions can be used on skin without the oil slick residue that an infused oil will leave behind. Their preparation is almost identical, and includes water, oil and an emulsifying agent that helps combine these two liquids.

Lotions have the thinner consistency of the two. This makes them suitable to be applied to large areas of skin, as in cases of sunburn. Because of their higher water content, lotions also tend to be more cooling and soothing. On the other hand, creams are semi-solid and easier to apply to small areas like cuts, scratches and small patches of eczema.

# OINTMENTS

Ointments are more solid than both creams and lotions, and are best used when you have a small area of skin to treat—as small as a mosquito bite or a cold sore—and want the remedy to sit on the skin and exert its action for a longer period of time, rather than to be quickly absorbed.

# INFUSIONS AND DECOCTIONS

Both of these words are basically just fancy naturopathic words for 'tea'. With that in mind, I want you to forget about the 'tea-bag-slapped-in-a-mug' kind of tea, and start to think 'therapeutics'. A properly brewed tea can be an easy and powerful medicine when used correctly, so don't underestimate how potent these two can be.

There are two basic ways to make a tea: infusions and decoctions. Infusions are best for leaves, flowers and any green part of the plant; decoctions are best for hard plant parts like seeds, bark and roots. For either type of tea you can use fresh or dried herbs. Imagine growing your favourite sleepy tea herb on your windowsill, and picking a handful just before bed for a fresh-leaf infusion that will send you off to a restful slumber. It couldn't be easier.

I remember that soon after I graduated, I blended a tea for my parents' insomnia. I researched it heavily, determined to get it right. I combined herbs from the Western, Ayurvedic and Chinese traditions, and crafted the tea blend to end all 'sleepy tea' blends. When I gave it to them and instructed them to enjoy two cups before bed, I think they thought it was 'a bit cute', so they humoured me and brewed a pot. After just one cup, my mum had to excuse herself and go straight to bed—she didn't even get around to pouring a second! The next night, my stepdad asked if I had 'any more of the stuff'. I've been making it for them ever since.

# BASIC INGREDIENTS AND EQUIPMENT

## HERBS

For fresh herbs, I always recommend that you grow your own if you can. It really is rewarding to pick them fresh from your own garden. There's little more thrilling than rushing out in the morning and seeing that the seeds you sowed have sprung into tiny

> There's little more thrilling than rushing out in the morning and seeing that the seeds you sowed have sprung into tiny little shoots.

little shoots, waiting to be nurtured into fully grown plants. This way, you can also ensure they are completely organic, meaning that no unwanted pesticides or herbicide residues end up in your otherwise pristine plant extracts. Plus you get a gold star for creating the remedy from start to finish.

If that's not an option, then get down to your nearest farmer's market and see what's on offer. Even your supermarket has a limited offering of herbs, so you may find just what you need there. If that's the case, I suggest that you give them a very thorough wash to get rid of any unwanted pesticides.

I will also be asking you to find some more obscure ingredients as we progress through the book. I will introduce you to some wonderful and strange herbs from around the world. Wherever possible I will use ingredients readily available in your local area, but sometimes there really is no substitute for the revered remedies of ancient medicinal traditions, and you need to head slightly further afield to make sure you're getting the

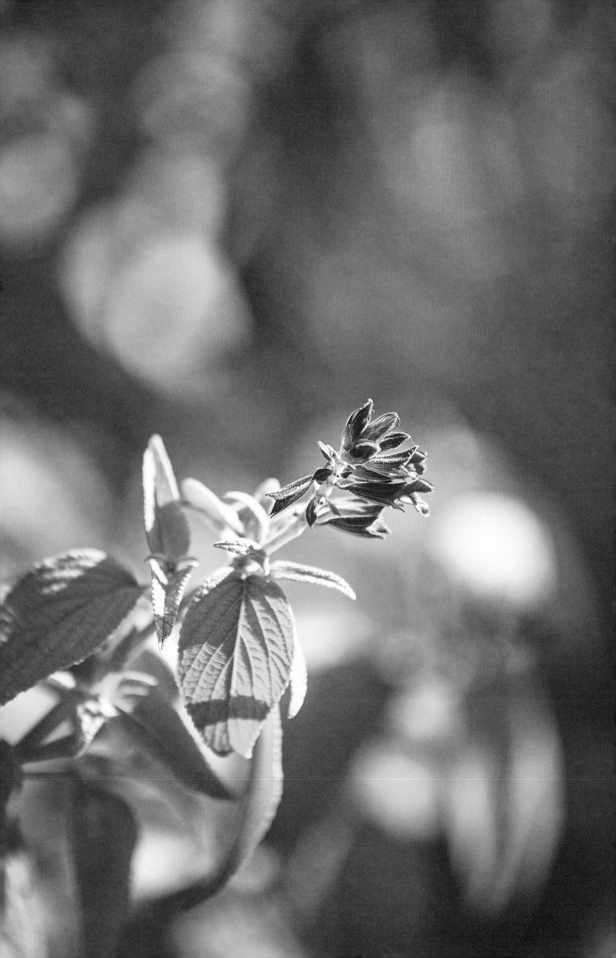

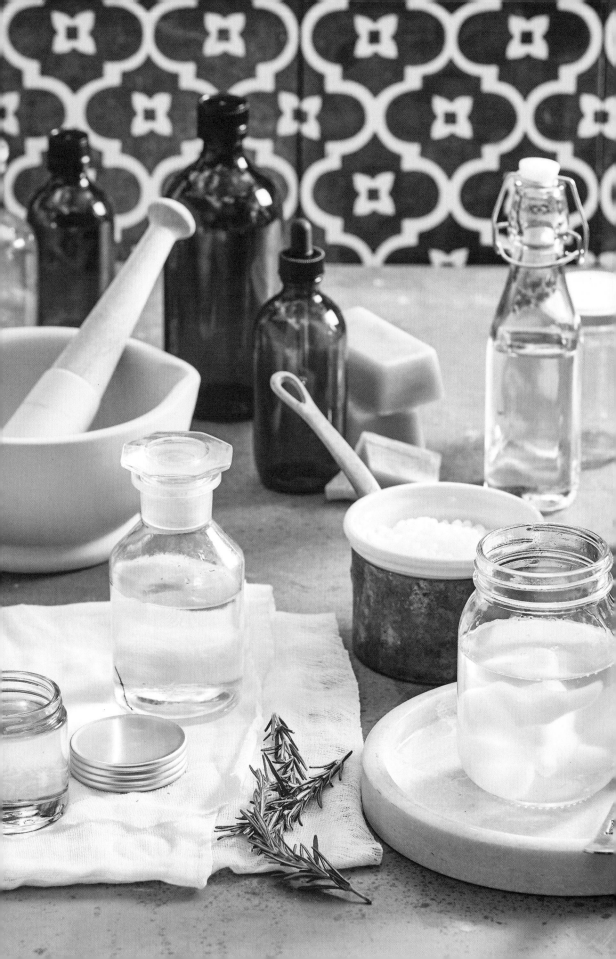

absolute best for your health. I doubt you'll find herbs like the Ayurvedic energy-balancing tonic ashwaganda down at the corner shop, so you may need to seek out a good health food store near you. If this is a confusing new experience for you, just ask the staff for help to find the dried herbs and loose-leaf teas. I've also provided a list of my favourite online stockists at the end of the book.

Of course, the herbs themselves are just the beginning! After you've chosen the right petals, seeds and leaves to transform into your remedy, you need to choose the right liquid, which we call a *menstruum*, to extract all the therapeutic compounds that give a plant its medicinal properties. The menstruum to use will depend on whether you're making a tincture, oil, tea or glycetract.

To become a fully-fledged herb nerd, you'll need the items below.

## COCONUT OIL

I frequently use this as an easy base for skin and hair oils. It's a quick and easy process to turn coconut oil into an infused oil, and you'll see it crop up in a few of my recipes.

You may have seen coconut oil sold in a liquid form, as well as the usual variety that is solid unless the weather gets warmer, in which case room temperatures often reach the point where it melts. Only the latter variety is true coconut oil. Perpetually liquid coconut oil is a refined product that has had the components with a higher melting point removed. One of those compounds is lauric acid, which is suggested to be antibacterial and therefore particularly beneficial when we're making an infused oil to be used on skin. When in doubt, always

choose the unrefined product: it will be solid in the cooler months, and liquefy as the temperatures warm up.

## SWEET ALMOND OIL

If your infused oil is going to be turned into a cream, you'll need an oil that, unlike coconut oil, stays liquid at room temperature. Sweet almond oil is my choice, as it's packed full of vitamin E, which promotes healthy skin healing. A good quality olive oil will do at a pinch.

## VODKA

Yep, I'm serious. We use vodka to turn our herbs into tinctures. The active compounds that give herbs their potency are, by nature, soluble to different degrees in ethanol (pure alcohol) and water. Clear spirits are a mixture of both, so you can be sure you're getting access to both the water- and alcohol-soluble goodness. Go organic if you can.

## VEGETABLE GLYCERINE

If you're making the remedy for your little ones, then I suggest using a mix of food-grade vegetable glycerine and water instead of vodka, for obvious reasons. Glycerine also makes for a thicker extract, so it works beautifully in remedies to soothe a dry, sore throat by coating the irritated tissue.

## EMULSIFYING WAX

When it comes to making creams and lotions, you need an emulsifying agent to stop the oil and water from separating. Wool, fat, egg yolk and all kinds of crazy things can be used as emulsifiers, depending on

**CLOCKWISE, FROM LEFT:** Mortar and pestle, amber glass bottles, beeswax, sweet almond oil, coconut oil, rosemary

whether you're adding oil to water or water to oil, but they are tricky to use and the process can be complex. Emulsifying wax is the easiest way to do this for a beginner, and leaves your remedy much less likely to split into its water and oil parts.

## BEESWAX

For ointments, beeswax helps as a setting agent. It comes in pellets or in solid blocks. Either will do, but if you opt for the latter make sure you've got a good set of knives—those blocks can be tough to chop through!

## COFFEE OR SPICE GRINDER

When dealing with dried herbs especially, breaking them down into a fine powder increases the surface area and improves extraction of the active compounds. You can use a mortar and pestle if you like, but a coffee or spice grinder is faster and much easier.

## CHEESECLOTH

Also called muslin, this coarsely woven fabric serves as a better strainer than your kitchen sieve. We use cheesecloth a lot to remove leftover herbs from our liquid remedies.

## JARS AND BOTTLES

Cold extractions, such as tinctures and infused oils, are done over two to three weeks in large jars, so these guys are essential. Amber glass is best, as it protects your medicines from damage caused by light. If you prefer clear glass then just ensure you keep the jars in a cool, dark cupboard. The same goes for bottles, which will be used to store the remedies. Depending on the remedy, you should get your hands on large bottles, small bottles and even spray bottles.

All glass used to store remedies needs sterilising before use.

## TO STERILISE GLASSWARE

This step is absolutely vital, as it makes sure there is no contamination in your remedies.

**Step 1** Pre-heat the oven to its lowest setting, which is usually around 70 degrees Celsius.

**Step 2** Place your glassware in the dishwasher and run at the hottest cycle. Alternatively, you can wash the glassware thoroughly with hot, soapy water. Rinse well to remove all detergent residue.

**Step 3** Place the glassware in a clean oven with the open end facing downwards. Leave for 20–30 minutes, or until they're bone dry. They're now ready to fill!

## OTHER EQUIPMENT

You'll also need all the kitchen basics: pots, pans, a blender, sieves, bowls, knives, measuring cups and jugs, chopping boards, kitchen thermometers—the lot! Food is medicine after all, so if you cook then you've most likely already got a lot of what you need.

CLOCKWISE, FROM LEFT: ginger, turmeric, pink sea salt

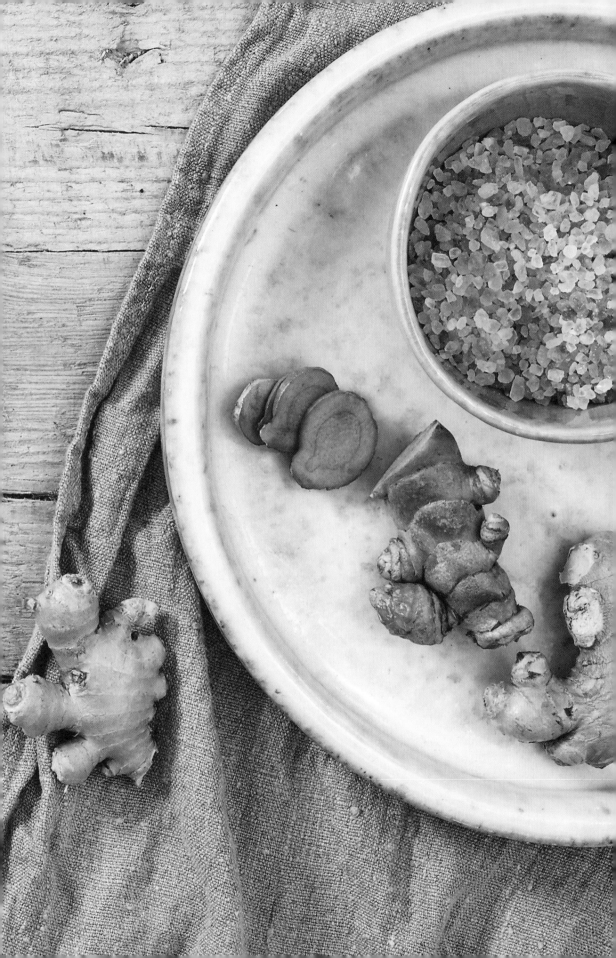

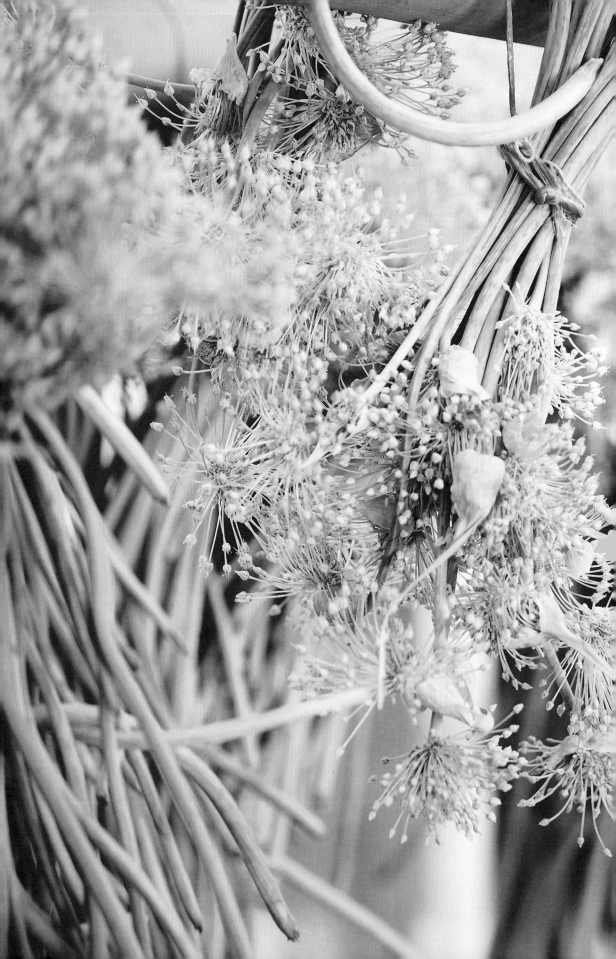

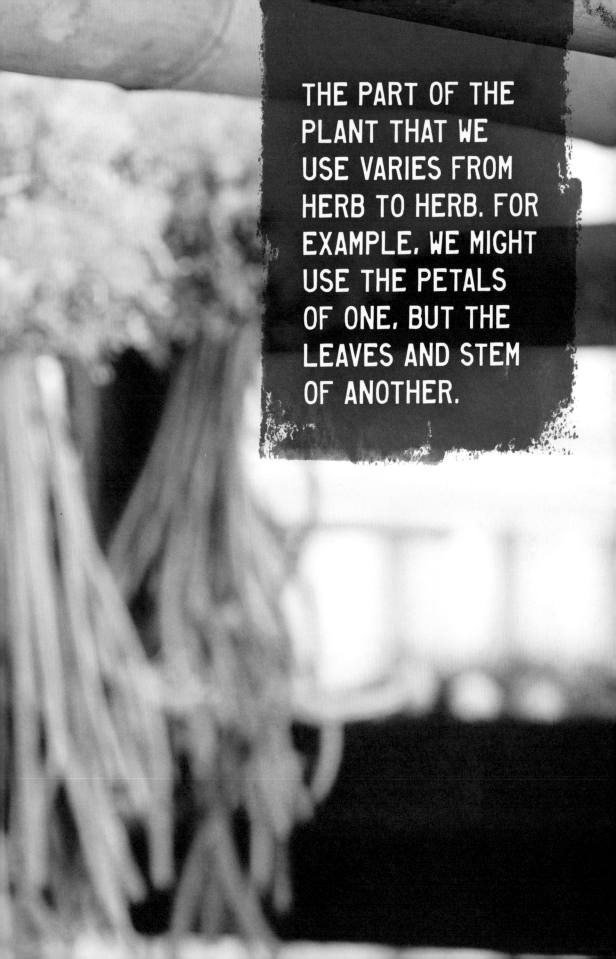

THE PART OF THE PLANT THAT WE USE VARIES FROM HERB TO HERB. FOR EXAMPLE, WE MIGHT USE THE PETALS OF ONE, BUT THE LEAVES AND STEM OF ANOTHER.

# GROWING A GARDEN APOTHECARY

*A guide to creating your own medicinal garden.*

**GROWING YOUR OWN** herbs is not an absolutely essential part of the process. A bundle of organic herbs from the farmer's market will do the job, or even your local supermarket might have a small selection—in which case you'll need to ensure you wash them even more thoroughly than usual to remove any chemical residue.

But if I have managed to convince you about the rewards of growing your own medicines, you might still be thinking of a few obstacles left to overcome. Maybe you don't think you have the space, time or skills? Or perhaps you imagine you need a sprawling backyard and a greenhouse or two? Not at all. Herbs are, for the most part, resilient little things. They don't need too much to thrive.

While I was lucky growing up on a farm that gave me all the space I could have wanted, I now live in an inner-city apartment far removed from the wide, open spaces of home. But that hasn't stopped me from having a garden. My miniscule balcony plays home to two rickety deck chairs from which to enjoy the summer sunshine, and surrounding the chairs are pots overflowing with greenery: an urban oasis.

You can create a garden sanctuary in even the tiniest of spaces, whether it's a balcony, a courtyard or even a windowsill—without spending a fortune. Small pots by a window are enough to get you started, and unless you keep your furniture on your ceiling, there's always space for a hanging basket or two. Below are a couple of my favourite space-saving garden designs that might help you to start your own herb garden.

> I was lucky growing up on a farm that gave me all the space I could have wanted.

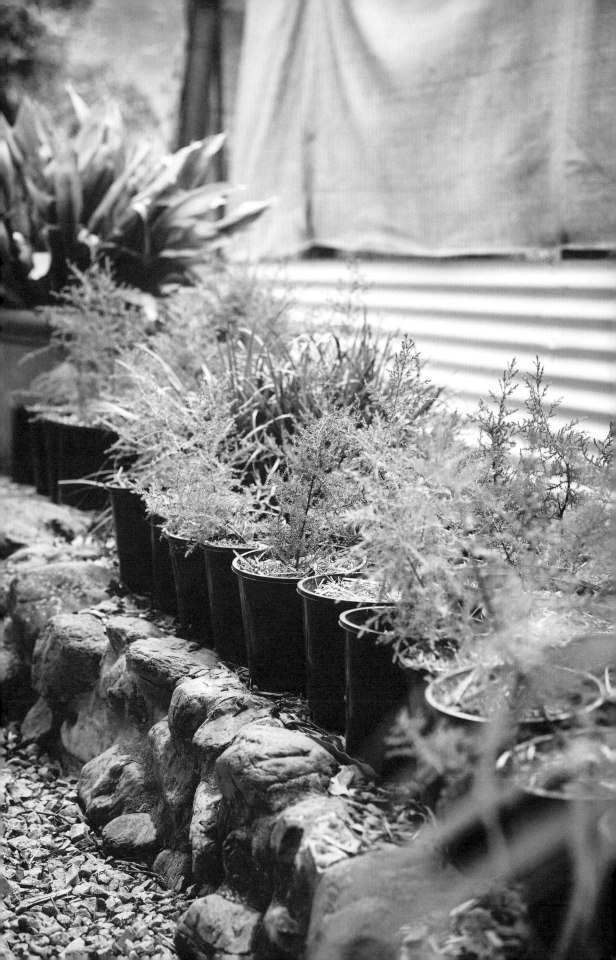

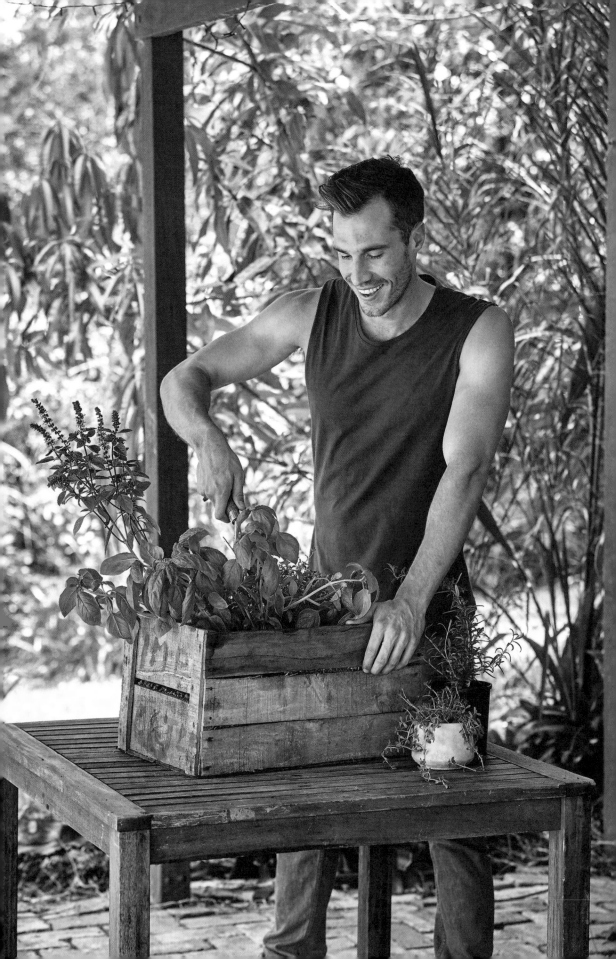

# APPLE CRATE PLANTERS

Turning old wooden boxes and crates into planter boxes couldn't be easier. I get mine from the generous greengrocer at my local market, but you can buy them online too. They come in all sizes, from teeny-tiny through to large enough to bathe in (not that I recommend that). Look for untreated pine to ensure you've not got nasties leaching into your soil.

## YOU WILL NEED

**A planter box**

**some builders plastic**

**scissors**

**a staple gun (or short nails/tacks and a hammer)**

**a Stanley knife**

**gravel, pea straw or lucerne hay**

**potting mix**

**organic compost**

**mulch**

**seeds or seedlings**

## HOW TO

**Step 1**  Measure the box, then cut a cross-shaped piece of builders plastic to line the inside. The plastic should be large enough to cover the base of the planter and run up all four sides.

**Step 2**  Secure the plastic in place along the base of the box with a staple gun, or with a hammer and short nails/tacks.

**Step 3**  At the opening of the box, secure the builders plastic in place just below where you intend to fill your planter with potting mix.

**Step 4**  With a Stanley knife, remove any excess plastic that rises out of the box. Fold any plastic above the staples back down over them and secure it in place. Pierce holes every couple of centimetres along the plastic lining the base of the planter to allow water to drain.

**Step 5**  Get your planter into position! Smaller boxes can be placed in hangers and attached to windowsills and balcony railings; larger boxes will need a little more space. I recommend raising them up slightly on a few bricks or spare pieces of timber, to allow water to flow out and away from the wood.

**Step 6**  Now you can begin to fill! Depending on the depth of your crate planter, you may want to line the bottom with gravel, pea straw or lucerne hay to improve drainage. Once that's in, it's just a matter of adding the potting mix and organic compost. As a general rule, I like to use about a half-and-half mix of the two, but check out the next chapter to determine exactly what your herbs of choice need, and whether they'll want mulch over them to keep the roots cool.

# Pallet Wall Gardens

The exact same principles can be applied to a wooden pallet as to an apple crate, but the end result is a stunning vertical garden that you can attach to any wall. Try to ensure the timber used for your vertical garden is untreated.

## YOU WILL NEED

**A wooden pallet**

**4 L-brackets to fit your choice of pallet**

**sandpaper**

**a hammer**

**builders plastic**

**a nail gun or hammer and short nails**

**a drill**

**potting mix**

**seedlings**

## HOW TO

**Step 1** Sand your pallet then hammer in any raised nails.

**Step 2** Cut and measure a piece of builders plastic to cover the back and three of the four sides. Be sure to leave plenty of excess plastic to cover the sides; I like about three times as much as I expect I'll need. The top and front face are going to be left uncovered. Using a nail gun or hammer and short nails, secure the plastic along the back of the pallet, keeping it taut.

**Step 3** Fold the plastic around the three sides that are to be covered, ensuring that no gaps are left for soil to fall out. Secure in place along the front edge, then fold back over the nails and around the back edge. Secure the plastic again along the back face, then trim any excess plastic. This ensures no rough edges of the plastic are on show, and looks much better.

**Step 4** Before you go ahead and fill the vertical garden, place it on the wall where it's going to be mounted and mark where the four L-brackets are going to go to hold it in place. Drill the L-brackets into the wall. Now it'll be easier to attach the planter to the brackets once it's full and much heavier.

**Step 5** Lay your pallet down, with the open face upwards. Start pouring in your potting mix, being sure to fill all the space between the slats. Every so often, you'll need to raise the pallet upright, shake the soil down into place and go again.

**Step 6** You need to plant the seedlings pretty densely to keep the soil from spilling out, and ensure the roots are secured between slats. Leave the pallet lying horizontal for a few weeks, watering daily to establish the plants.

**Step 7** Once the roots have taken hold and the soil is less likely to fall out, you can raise the garden upright and, with help, attach it to the wall.

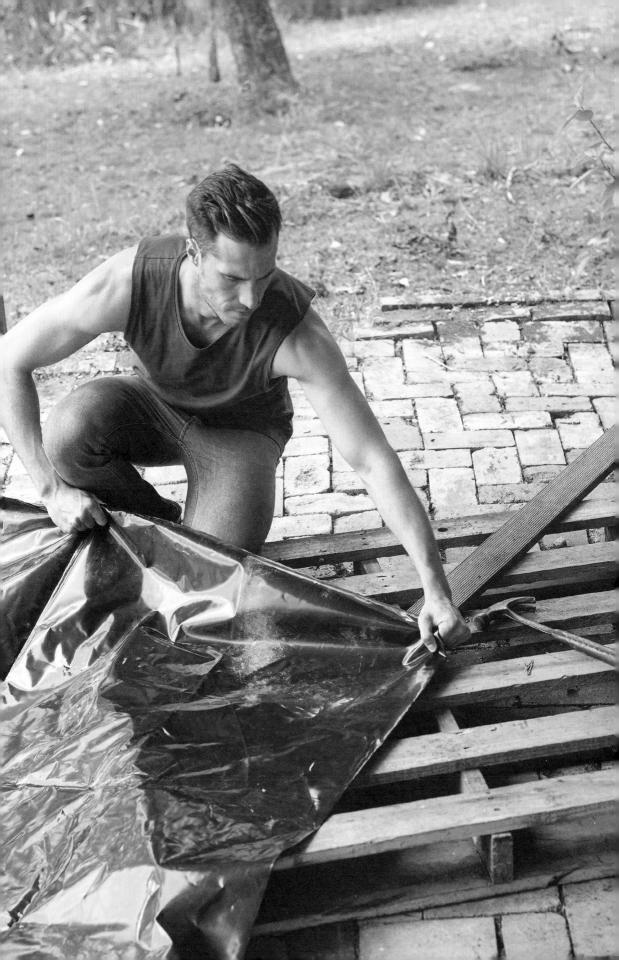

# WHAT SHALL I GROW?

'But I'd kill a cactus!' you say? Rubbish. It's a myth that you need to be born with a green thumb to be able to grow a garden. I'm testament to that: I started my first ever herb and veggie garden back when I was still shorter than the garden rake, and even I managed to keep things alive.

Start simple: pick an ailment that bothers you most, and grow a handful of herbs to tackle that. A single pot or planter box is enough if you've got limited space, although I have a sneaking suspicion that once you get going, you won't want to stop.

If you're wondering which herbs to grow for what ailment, in this chapter I've listed some of my favourite plants to grow and how to do it. So now you can get your garden apothecary started, regardless of your alleged plant murderer status!

## ALOE VERA (ALOE BARBADENSIS)
—Grow me to soothe sunburn

**What is it?**
You will have noticed green bottles of gel in the sunscreen section of your local pharmacist. The aloe vera gel in pure form is derived from a pretty succulent and is widely used to soothe skin. It can also be taken internally to exert its healing actions on the gut.

**Planting**
**Season** It's best to buy an existing plant and take good care of it, rather than try to grow it from scratch.
**Soil** Give your aloe a nice free-draining soil.
**Sunlight** Picture where you would imagine aloe growing as a native plant. Is it somewhere sunny, rugged and hot? Use that as a guide for where you place your aloe: it likes full sun.

**Care**
As you might expect, aloe vera likes warm weather. If you live somewhere that suffers frosts, keep your plant indoors by a window, or in a greenhouse. Apart from that, aloe doesn't demand much attention. For the most part it thrives on neglect!

**When to harvest**
Cut off the oldest, largest leaves when you need them.

**How do I use it?**
Slice the leaf open by removing the 'flatter' side with a sharp knife. You should now have a long trough of beautiful gel in front of you, ready to be scooped out and used. Be careful not to use any of the green juice or fibrous

Start simple: pick an ailment that bothers you most, and grow a handful of herbs to tackle that.

bits, which in fact can be irritating to the skin for a small number of people. Apply the pure gel directly to sunburn, or blend into a green smoothie like the one on page 136.

## BRAHMI (BACOPA MONNIERI)
—*Grow me to aid memory*

**What is it?**
Okay, so this low-lying creeper is a little on the fancier side, being borrowed from the Ayurvedic tradition of medicine. It isn't necessarily something you will see at every nursery, but if you can get your hands on it then you are in luck: brahmi is the best memory and cognition tonic around.

**Planting**
**Season** Plant your brahmi in spring and summer.
**Soil** It often lives alongside bodies of water, so at home you should grow it in moist, richly fertilised soil.
**Sunlight** This herb, direct from India and Sri Lanka, likes part-shade to full shade.

**Care**
Brahmi likes to be kept nice and wet, so don't let the roots dry out. Fertilise regularly—a liquid seaweed fertiliser works best—and in colder months make sure you move your plant somewhere warm.

**When to harvest**
Once your creeper is established, you can pick the leaves whenever you like.

**How do I use it?**
Brahmi can be made as an infusion, but I prefer to make a big bottle of the tincture (see page 54 for how to make tinctures) by combining it with ginkgo and gotu kola for a memory tonic. Three teaspoons with breakfast and lunch is the best way to dose this mix, and you'll really start to see results after a few weeks of regular use.

## CALENDULA (CALENDULA OFFICINALIS)
—*Grow me for skin health*

**What is it?**
A member of the daisy family, calendulas are going to be your little darlings when it comes to happy skin. Bright orange in appearance, their petals promote skin healing. It's a miracle herb for conditions like eczema.

**Planting**
**Season** If using seed, start in containers inside at the very start of spring. If you're saving yourself that hassle and using existing plants, wait until later in the season when frosts are less likely before you find them a home outside.
**Soil** Calendulas like medium soil with good drainage, and do well in pots.
**Sunlight** Place your calendulas where they will get plenty of sun in the mornings.

**Care**
Calendulas like to stay relatively cool but with plenty of sunlight, so add a layer of mulch to your soil so it doesn't dry out and fry the roots. Pulling off the flower heads may seem cruel, but doing it regularly encourages new ones to grow, meaning that you get lots more 'bang for your buck'.

**When to harvest**
A good calendula plant will provide flowers from spring right through until the end of autumn—and sometimes beyond if you're lucky!

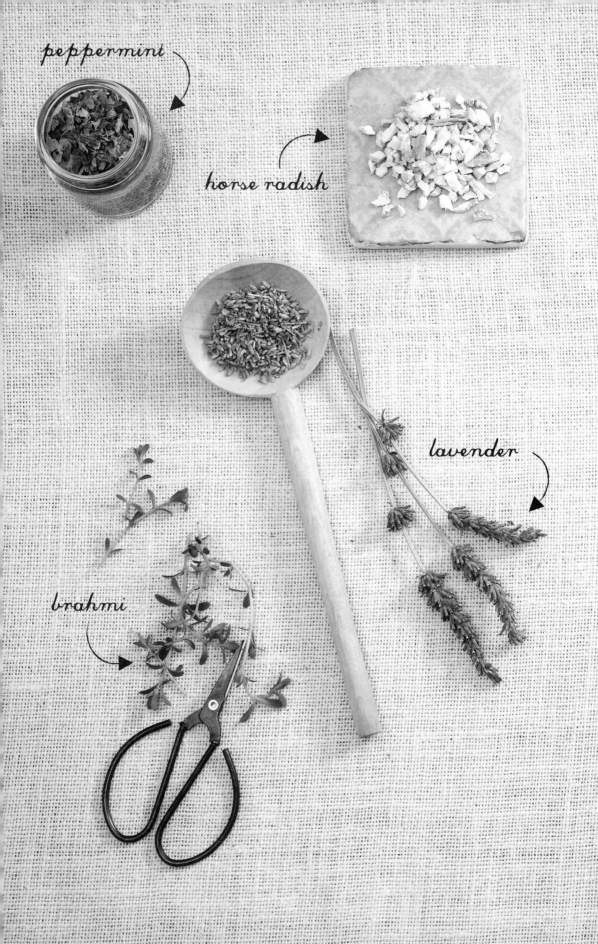

*peppermint*

*horse radish*

*lavender*

*brahmi*

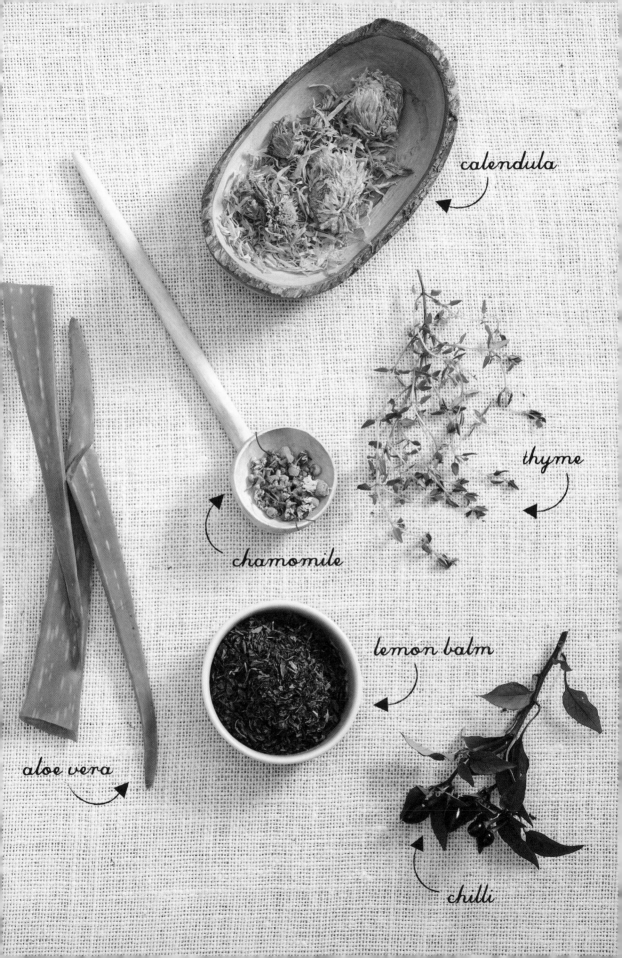

calendula

thyme

chamomile

aloe vera

lemon balm

chilli

## How do I use it?

It makes sense, since you'll be picking the calendula flowers as often as you can, to dry them out until you need them. Although whole flower heads can be dried, I find it easiest for beginners to remove the petals and just dry those—after all, that's where all the goodness is. Drying the whole thing can be difficult because they retain moisture, giving mould a chance to take hold. See page 45 for drying instructions. Once dry, you can store your petals in a jar, ready to turn into oils (see page 60) or to sprinkle on salads.

## CHILLI (CAPSICUM SPP.)
*—Grow me for weight loss*

### What is it?

The heat in chilli is a dead giveaway of its medicinal properties: it fires up metabolism and warms a sluggish body.

### Planting

**Season** Like with aloe vera, chillies are happiest in the warmer months. Pick up an existing plant and pop it in a larger pot, so that you can give it sunshine in summer, but bring it inside to protect it from frosts when it gets cold.
**Soil** Load the pot up with a medium soil.
**Sunlight** Place your chilli plant in full sun. I like to think of the plant absorbing all the heat and transferring it to the fruit.

### Care

Like tomatoes—if you've ever grown them—chillies can be susceptible to pesky little nematodes, so make sure you use fresh potting mix whenever you transplant one. Also, don't grow chillies in the same place over and over; good crop rotation practices ensure healthier plants. Don't overfertilise your chillies, or you'll get lots of foliage instead of fruit. Water the plant regularly, but with only a little water at a time.

### When to harvest

Your plant will bear the most fruit in the summer months, which is when to pick them.

### How do I use it?

Unless you're adding them directly to your meals, dried chillies are easier to work with. Hang them in a warm, dry place until ready. You can make a delicious chilli oil with garlic, ginger and olive oil, which works in soups and stews in the winter months when your plant won't be fruiting.

## GERMAN CHAMOMILE (MATRICARIA RECUTITA)
*—Grow me for sleep*

### What is it?

Most of us only know chamomile as something that comes in a tea bag, often filled with decaying grey twigs. The vibrant yellow of the fresh flower is a hundred times better. Chamomile is another member of the daisy family and has traditionally been used to bring on sleep. It is also a gentle anti-inflammatory perfectly suited for external use on kids' sensitive skin. If the floral taste reminds you too much of Grandma's house, check out lemon balm as a substitute.

### Planting

**Season** Plant in spring by dropping the seeds directly on top of the soil, pressing down and watering them in. Don't cover the seeds, as they need a decent amount of sunlight to sprout. Keep in mind that the seeds are tiny, so to get good distribution I like to bulk them up with sand and sprinkle the mix over the area you plan to grow them. Otherwise it's very easy to get overzealous and dump all the seeds in one spot.

**Soil** Chamomile likes light, sandy soil with good drainage.

**Sunlight** Plant in a sunny position—at most it will tolerate partial shade.

## Care

Like many herbs, chamomile is deceptively hardy. Tough love is the name of the game here, so only water it every second or third day, and never let the soil get soggy. Avoid too much fertiliser, as that may cause fast growth of the foliage, but a disappointing number of flowers. Keep the area free of weeds and after 2 to 4 weeks, thin the plants out to give them room to grow.

## When to harvest

Chamomile is usually ready to harvest a few months after being planted. Pick the flower heads as needed, or dry them for future use (see page 45).

## How do I use it?

An infusion of chamomile tea can be made by taking three teaspoons of the fresh flowers and steeping them in a mug of hot water for 5 minutes. Consider combining chamomile with lemon balm and mint for a brew that is both good for digestion and calms a frazzled nervous system. It's the perfect night-time infusion!

Chamomile also makes a killer infused oil for skin and is gentler than something like calendula. It's perfect for sensitive skin, especially for the younger family members.

# HORSERADISH (AMORACIA RUSTICANA)
*—Grow me to alleviate a cold*

## What is it?

Who knew that horseradish wasn't just an obscure jar hanging about in the back of the fridge? This root vegetable is actually a seriously powerful decongestant, used to blast open stuffy sinuses, and it ranks as one of the easiest edible plants to grow.

## Planting

**Season** Plant in either early autumn or spring from a root cutting. Dig a deep hole, add plenty of compost, then plant the root about 30 centimetres below the surface before filling it in.

**Soil** Any, as long as it isn't consistently waterlogged.

**Sunlight** Plant horseradish in full sun if you can, or at the very least give it direct sunlight for half the day.

## Care

Plant it, bury it, ignore it: that's how easy it is with horseradish. Water it whenever you water the rest of your garden, but don't overdo it; soggy soil is the one thing horseradish can't handle.

## When to harvest

You will need to leave it at least a year until your horseradish is ready to harvest. Carefully dig the root up, and remove it completely. Wash it well and slice off a small piece to replant.

## How do I use it?

You can make a tincture if you're brave (see page 54) but I prefer to incorporate this medicine into my winter meals. Its kick can be softened by grating it up and combining it with a fatty dairy product, like softened butter or crème fraiche.

## LAVENDER (LAVANDULA ANGUSTIFOLIA)
*—Grow me to relieve anxiety*

### What is it?
I'm often asked what my favourite herb is. After the initial recoil that follows being asked to choose between my children, my answer is always lavender. Quite apart from the fact that it conjures up images of rolling fields in the south of France, lavender is known to lift mood and soothe anxiety.

### Planting
**Season** Let's face it: not many of us have time to grow a lavender plant from scratch. Instead, buy a potted plant and transplant it to a larger container in spring or autumn, or buy a few and start a hedge!
**Soil** Lavender wants a medium soil with good drainage.
**Sunlight** Full sun will give the best lavender plants, rich in the essential oils that give it its familiar scent.

### Care
Young plants need daily watering through their first summer, but otherwise lavender is pretty tough and can look after itself. If you see the leaves starting to turn yellow, it's a good sign that it's thirsty. In terms of pruning, you'll want to give it a good trim each year, but not into old wood.

### When to harvest
Once lavender is established, you can pick a few flower heads as you need them. You can also dry the flowers (see page 45), then crumble the flowers up for inclusion into dried tea blends.

### How do I use it?
In an infusion (see page 63) lavender combines beautifully with another anti-anxiety herb, passionflower. You can also just crush a few flower heads and place them under your pillowcase; lavender contains an oil called linalool that has been shown to reduce an anxious heart rate by inhalation alone!

## LEMON BALM (MELISSA OFFICINALIS)
*—Grow me to alleviate stress*

### What is it?
Lemon balm, sometimes called Melissa, is mint's relaxing cousin. Lemon balm is used to reduce anxiety and promote restfulness, so can indeed be used in place of chamomile if you prefer its clean, citrus-like taste.

### Planting
**Season** Plant the seed or seedlings in spring.
**Soil** Lemon balm likes a rich, well-drained soil, and like others of its family will take over if you're not careful, so consider keeping it in a pot.
**Sunlight** Full sun will work for lemon balm in most locations, but consider placing it in partial shade if you live somewhere hot.

### Care
Water daily and keep a layer of mulch over the soil to keep it from drying out. If you have good quality soil, then you shouldn't need to fertilise. In fact, too much fertiliser and you might find that your lemon balm isn't as aromatic. If not pruned every now and again, lemon balm has the potential to get out of hand.

**When to harvest**

Harvest throughout the summer, picking the leaves as required.

**How do I use it?**

Lemon balm has another cute nickname: herbal valium. Its sedative actions are particularly potent when combined with lavender in a tea, or with valerian and hops in a tincture. Besides its bedtime benefits, lemon balm has a reputation as being a natural mosquito repellent, so crush it and rub on any exposed skin while you're out in the garden—you'll smell great too!

## PEPPERMINT (MENTHA PIPERITA)
*—Grow me to help bloating*

**What is it?**

Tummy troubles? Peppermint is the answer. It's a perfect 'after dinner' tea, acting as a *carminative* herb, meaning that it reduces bloating and indigestion. And the best news? It's so easy to grow that you may actually find the biggest difficulty is stopping it from taking over!

**Planting**

**Season** Grab a seedling from your local nursery in spring, and make sure you've got plenty of room for it to grow when you get it home. If you're a garden pro, you can also grow peppermint from a cutting.

**Soil** Peppermint likes constant water, so pick a patch of soil that is nice and moist.

**Sunlight** It's not as fussy as other plants, but I would recommend aiming for partial shade.

**Care**

I like to grow peppermint—and indeed all kinds of mint—in a pot or planter box. That stops it from taking over the garden, which it will do if given the chance. Water daily and ensure it isn't left in blistering heat.

**When to harvest**

You can harvest your peppermint leaves by pinching them from the stalk whenever you want, but ensure you never take more than one-third of the leaves, and allow them to grow back before you take more. If you have cold winters, harvest as much as you can as everything above ground will die off in the cold, then regenerate in the warmer months.

**How do I use it?**

A handful of fresh peppermint leaves steeped in hot water makes an excellent remedy for a bloated tummy. Crushing the leaves in your hands and inhaling stimulates a tired mind and banishes brain fog too!

## THYME (THYMUS VULGARIS)
*—Grow me to ward off infections*

**What is it?**

This resilient herb is one of nature's best antibacterial offerings, so keep lots of it on hand in winter for when infections attack.

Let me save you the trouble; thyme tincture tastes awful

### Planting

**Season** Thyme is best planted from a seedling in spring, but you can get away with planting it any time of the year.
**Soil** Lighter, well-draining soils are best for thyme.
**Sunlight** Thyme, like me, is a sun-lover. Give it full sunlight.

### Care

Thankfully, thyme is another herb that likes to be ignored, making it perfect for the herb nerd just starting out. This wild-child is best left alone to do its own thing, so water sparingly. A little compost once a year, in spring, doesn't go astray.

### When to harvest

Don't go too hard on harvesting your thyme in the first year, as this woody perennial won't grow back as quickly as something like mint. Its oils are most potent in summertime, so pick sprigs then and hang them to dry for winter. See page 45 for more drying tips.

### How do I use it?

Let me save you the trouble: thyme tinctures taste awful. Just don't do it. I also don't think the teas are particularly palatable, so instead extract the active compounds in a jar of apple cider vinegar, crushed garlic and sage. After two weeks, strain and keep the liquid as a gargle for sore throats. Brush your teeth after each use, as vinegar is acidic and can damage enamel if you don't rinse it off.

# A NOTE ON THE DAISY FAMILY

The daisy family of plants, more correctly known as the Asteraceae family, can cause contact dermatitis and other allergic symptoms in susceptible individuals. It affects middle-aged and elderly adults most frequently, and is worse in summer months. Although uncommon, it is worth noting in case you find you develop skin irritation from growing, handling or using remedies that contain this family. Members of the Asteraceae family used in this book include German chamomile, calendula, dandelion, echinacea and feverfew. Discontinue use if you suspect you may be allergic.

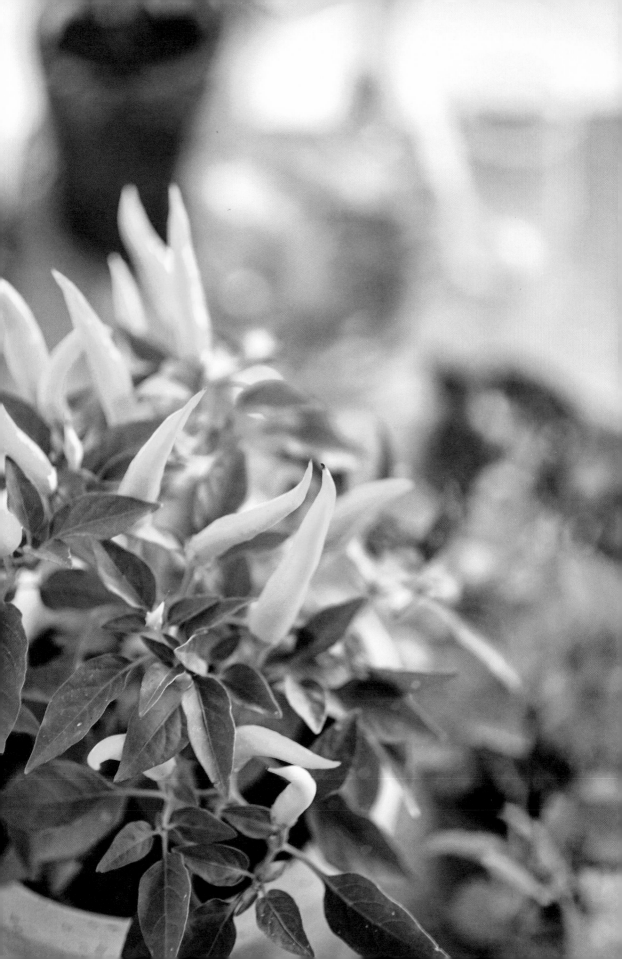

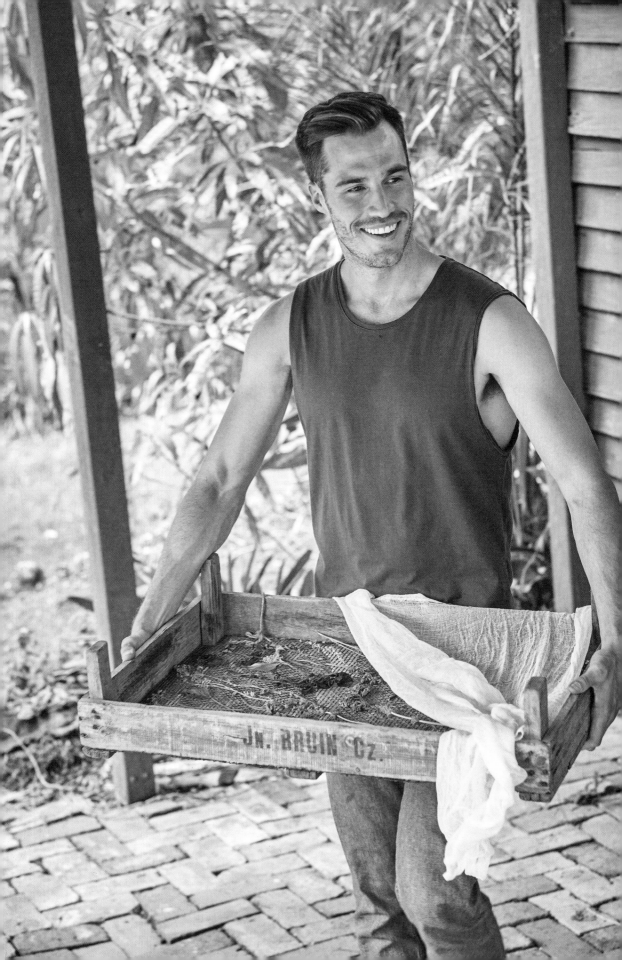

# DRYING YOUR OWN HERBS

Fresh herbs are great when it comes to food as medicine or for use in fresh teas, but you can make your tinctures even stronger by drying the plant materials first. Drying your herbs removes the water content, concentrating the active compounds in the process. It also prolongs their shelf life by up to a year, so that you can have access to all kinds of herbal medicine year round, without the environmental and health concerns of using produce out of season.

## YOU WILL NEED

**A flywire frame**

**fresh herbs**

**paper towel**

**one large sheet of cheesecloth**

**bulldog clips**

**clothes horse**

## HOW TO

**Step 1** Take an old flywire frame and give it a good clean in soapy water, then rinse. Leave to dry, as you don't want any excess moisture on it when it comes time to dry your herbs.

**Step 2** Wash your freshly harvested herbs, remove excess water with paper towel and then scatter over the flywire in a single layer. Leave space between them and avoid clumping so as to maximise airflow. The smaller the pieces are, and the more they are spread out, the faster they'll dry. Pull any petals from the flower heads and let them dry individually. With roots and barks, break or slice them up before drying.

**Step 3** Cover with a piece of cheesecloth, and secure it in place with bulldog clips.

**Step 4** You'll need to raise your drying rack up off the ground, so a clothes horse does a fine job, especially if you have multiple racks on the go at once.

**Step 5** Leave your herbs to dry in a warm, well-ventilated place away from direct sunlight. If the temperature is between 25–35 degrees Celsius, your herbs should be ready to store in glass jars after about a week. Delicate herbs might be ready in as little as three days, and others will require ten days or more. For leaves, petals and stems, you'll know they're dry when you can crumble them in your hand.

If the drying process seems a little arduous, you can find suppliers of affordable dried herbs who will deliver to your door on page 174 or head down to the health food store and see what loose-leaf teas they have in stock.

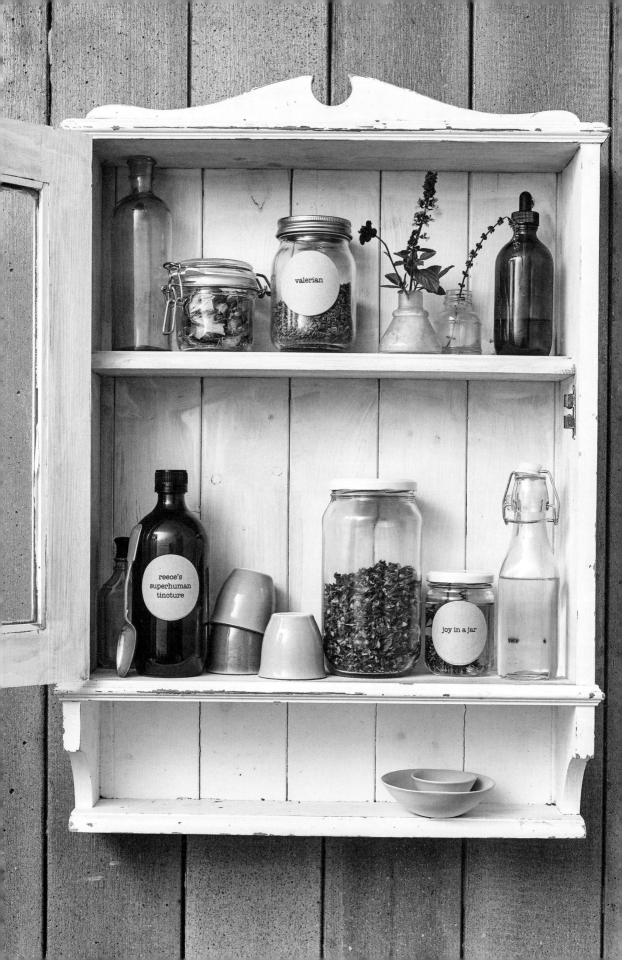

# STOCKING THE PANTRY

## My favourite ingredients to have on hand

**LOOK AT THAT** spice rack. Hiding among the barely touched jars lie potent natural medicines, just waiting to be plucked from the shelf so they can show off their health benefits. See that bottle of fennel seeds you bought, used once, and then forgot about? Crack it open again and make a decoction. Now add a handful of peppermint from the garden and—voila—you've got a tea to banish the bloat after a big meal. And the cinnamon you bought when you went through that baking phase? Blend a pinch or two into your morning smoothie to help keep sweet cravings at bay for the rest of the day.

Your local farmer's market can become your pharmacy, and your pantry can morph into a medicine cabinet, with a little knowledge of which humble ingredients have a physiological effect on the body. I've laid out ten of my must-haves to make it easy for you to get started.

## DANDELION

### WHAT IS IT?

Like so many of our herbal heroes, dandelion is actually considered a weed! You've probably got plenty of it growing in your backyard, but since it's easily confused with another herb called cat's ear, I don't recommend that you play botanist and forage for your own. We use two parts of the plant in herbal medicine: the green leaves stimulate digestion, and the root is used for liver complaints.

### WHAT CAN I USE IT FOR?

Loss of appetite, constipation.

### HOW DO I USE IT?

The green leaves are best incorporated into a salad or juice, but be warned that they are very bitter and you may need to blend them with some less intense greens such as spinach or even wild lettuce. The root can be bought roasted and makes a great caffeine-free alternative to coffee.

### WHERE CAN I FIND IT?

You may need to become best friends with your local veggie growers to see if they can bring you some dandelion greens, but the roasted root is much easier to find in health food stores. I recommend avoiding the instant formulas sold in some supermarkets, and sticking to a wholefood option.

# ELDERFLOWER

## WHAT IS IT?

Elderflowers are tiny creamy-white flowers that grow on elder trees in big clusters called umbels. They appear just when we need them, when allergies hit in springtime.

## WHAT CAN I USE IT FOR?

Hayfever, allergies, colds and to help children with a runny nose.

## HOW DO I USE IT?

Since elderflower is one of our tastiest herbal medicines, I like to turn it into a cordial with rice malt syrup, water, lemons and oranges. Mix the cordial through sparkling water when the allergies hit and you've got one delicious medicine. If that's all too much effort, it can be brewed as a simple infusion.

## WHERE CAN I FIND IT?

In spring, elder trees fill the air with the most amazing scent, and that's the time to pick the umbels before they turn bitter. If you don't have an elder tree in your area, the dried flowers are sold as a tea in health food stores.

# FENNEL SEED

## WHAT IS IT?

Fennel is a small, elongated seed that comes from a plant from the same family as the carrot. It tastes a bit like aniseed, and in traditional medicine is regarded as a *carminative* and *spasmolytic*. That means that, along with fresh peppermint from your garden, it's about to become your strongest ally when it comes to the battle of the bloat; the oils in fennel relax muscles in the gut and make for easier digestion.

## WHAT CAN I USE IT FOR?

Irritable Bowel Syndrome (IBS), bloating, cramps, flatulence.

## HOW DO I USE IT?

Buy whole seeds, then grind them with either a mortar and pestle or a spice grinder before you use them, so as to maximise their effect. Being a hardened, fibrous part of the plant, they'll need to be decocted (see page 63) for 10 minutes.

## WHERE CAN I FIND IT?

Fennel seeds are readily available in supermarkets, among the dried herbs and spices.

# GARLIC

## WHAT IS IT?

Garlic bulbs really are a gift from nature. Known to boost immunity, kill off bad bugs and even help lower 'bad cholesterol', garlic is a tonic we should all be on. Keep the parsley within reach though, and munch on a handful afterwards to ward off garlic breath.

## WHAT CAN I USE IT FOR?

Maintaining healthy cholesterol and lipid levels, boosting immunity in winter and fighting off colds.

## HOW DO I USE IT?

Garlic is a classic example of food as medicine, and should be combined with thyme in soups and broths throughout the winter months. As a quick remedy, I like to crush enough bulbs to fill a small jar, then pour over apple cider vinegar. Leave the jar at room temperature for a week or two to remove some of the intense flavour, then strain. In a new jar, mix the garlic with manuka honey. I have a teaspoon of this every morning in winter to keep my immune system ticking. Sensitive tummies can sometimes find this a bit much, so avoid using it this way with kids or if you know you're prone to a sore stomach.

## WHERE CAN I FIND IT?

I'm not a fan of dried garlic or garlic powders, so dodge the aisles of your supermarket and pick up the fresh stuff in the fruit and veggie section instead. I prefer the purple bulbs over the white ones, which have often been bleached.

# GINGER

## WHAT IS IT?

Like its colourful cousin turmeric, ginger acts as an anti-inflammatory. It's also my absolute favourite option when feeling nauseous. In traditional Chinese medicine, ginger is used to warm a cold body, and so it is a great tea to sip on during cooler weather.

## WHAT CAN I USE IT FOR?

Bloating, colds, nausea, period pain, motion sickness and even hangovers.

## HOW DO I USE IT?

A simple infusion is the easiest way to use ginger, and having it as a steaming mug of tea maximises its heating effect on the body. Fresh is best, so take a rhizome, then peel and grate three teaspoons to add to boiled water.

## WHERE CAN I FIND IT?

Supermarkets, farmers' markets and greengrocers all sell fresh ginger.

# GREEN TEA

## WHAT IS IT?

Green tea is produced from the leaves of the same plant as black tea, *Camellia sinensis*, but is less processed. It's full of catechins, which have been rigorously tested in clinical trials to show their antioxidant and immune-stimulating effects. Other compounds called xanthines have given green tea a reputation as a metabolism-booster and weight loss aid. As if all that wasn't enough to land it a permanent spot in your pantry, it's also strongly antibacterial. As a teenager, I spent a lot of time ridding myself of pubescent pimples with a damp green tea bag—true story!

### WHAT CAN I USE IT FOR?

Colds and flu, weight loss, fatigue, acne.

### HOW DO I USE IT?

If it's not broken, don't fix it; green tea is still best consumed as an infusion two or three times a day. To clean your skin, brew a cup of tea and then remove the tea bag. Leave it to cool (we don't want to apply a hot tea bag to skin—ouch!) and then dab the damp tea bag onto your skin.

### WHERE CAN I FIND IT?

Green tea is widely available in supermarkets, both as tea bags and loose-leaf varieties.

# LICORICE

### WHAT IS IT?

Before you get too excited, I'm not giving you the all clear to jump into the sweets aisle. Licorice root was once used to flavour confectionery, but has mostly been abandoned now in favour of artificial alternatives. The root itself though is an incredible tonic, and herbalists use it to aid in recovery from periods of intense stress, both physical and emotional.

### WHAT CAN I USE IT FOR?

Recovery and adaptation to stress, and sore throats. Avoid licorice if you may have high blood pressure, and check with your doctor first.

### HOW DO I USE IT?

Licorice tea is my favourite, especially when combined with a few fresh lavender heads to calm anxious thoughts. If you're using it for a sore throat, a glycetract is easy to make, and you'll have a remedy that provides soothing relief to dry, irritated tissue; see page 149 to learn how.

### WHERE CAN I FIND IT?

You'll need to head to a health food store to find licorice root, and I recommend that you dodge the second-rate tea bags and get good quality loose-leaf product instead.

# OATS

### WHAT IS IT?

'Oats aren't a herbal medicine!' I hear you cry, and maybe you're right, but they are such a medicinally powerful food that I couldn't leave them out. The fibres in oats bind to excess cholesterol in the gut and help lower 'bad cholesterol'. They also leave skin feeling silky smooth when used in external preparations.

### WHAT CAN I USE IT FOR?

Maintaining healthy blood cholesterol and lipids, and eczema.

### HOW DO I USE IT?

Don't bother trying to turn oats into a tincture because the best way is still to have them for breakfast—in porridge, raw muesli or as an addition to your morning smoothie.

### WHERE CAN I FIND IT?

When you get to the cereal aisle of the supermarket, avoid the 'instant oats' and instead pick up a bag of whole rolled oats in all their glory.

# TURMERIC

### WHAT IS IT?

Turmeric really is the king of anti-inflammatories. It contains a little something called *curcumin*, which is believed to work in the same way as pharmaceutical anti-inflammatories. And the good news? It doesn't have the nasty side effects, leaving your gut lining healthy and happy.

### WHAT CAN I USE IT FOR?

Irritable bowel syndrome (IBS), arthritis and joint pain.

### HOW DO I USE IT?

Turmeric has an earthy flavour that lends itself to curries and rice dishes, so load up your Asian meals with this anti-inflammatory powerhouse. Curcumin is a large molecule and doesn't readily pass into the bloodstream, but there's a little secret to increase its absorption: add a pinch of black pepper. Prefer something sweeter? Turmeric is also cropping up in chai tea recipes, and combines well with other spices and honey.

### WHERE CAN I FIND IT?

Fresh turmeric looks like a smaller ginger rhizome—and indeed, they are related. If you snap it open, you'll find the inside is bright orange. You might need to head to a farmer's market or greengrocer to find it fresh, but dried turmeric is readily available in supermarkets as a yellow powder. The studies suggest that the dried form is still pretty potent, so powdered turmeric is still a great starting point for the brand new herb nerd.

# VALERIAN

### WHAT IS IT?

Valerian root was my first introduction to herbal medicine, when I decided to take a natural sleep aid on a long-haul flight. It was a big mistake opening the tincture inside the plane; it didn't take long for valerian's tell-tale old sock smell to fill the cabin.

### WHAT CAN I USE IT FOR?

Insomnia, mild anxiety.

### HOW DO I USE IT?

Since valerian contains a lot of active compounds that are soluble in fat but not water, making a decoction of this herb seems kind of pointless. Instead, take Mum's advice and have a glass of warm milk before bed. Use full-cream dairy milk or, if you can't have dairy, then use your favourite alternative with some coconut oil stirred through. Bring the milk to a boil, add two teaspoons of finely chopped valerian root and leave to simmer for 10 minutes. Strain, add some honey or a natural sugar alternative like stevia and sip yourself to sleep.

### WHERE CAN I FIND IT?

Growing valerian is an option, but it takes a few years to grow to a decent size, and is best harvested in winter. Given that insomnia can strike year-round, I like to pick up some dried valerian root from my health food store so that it's always on hand.

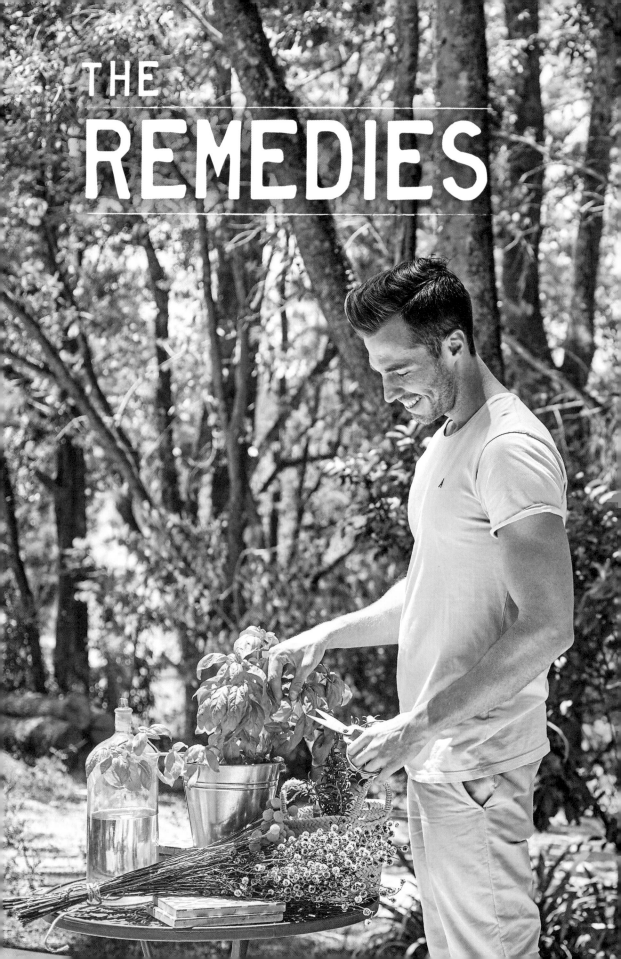

# THE REMEDIES

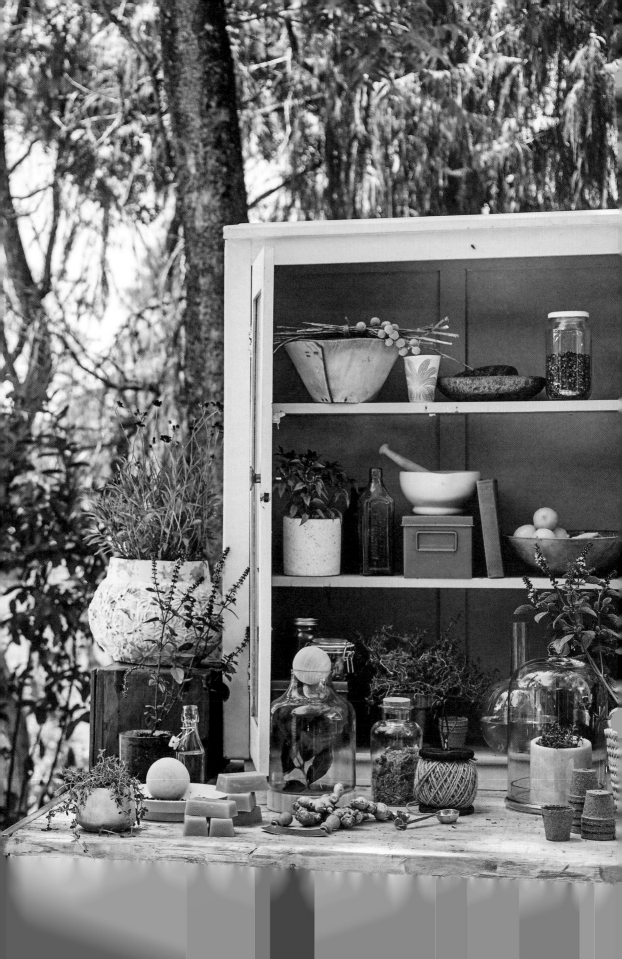

# BASIC TECHNIQUES

*For tinctures, oils, infusions and decoctions*

**RATHER THAN A** recipe book, I want you to think of this as a remedy book. Some creations in the coming chapters are for yummy treats and pantry staples; others are full-blown, palate-blasting tinctures and tonics that are far more medicinal than they are mouth-watering. What they all have in common is that they deliver a whopping great hit of therapeutic effect and get a big naturopathic tick of approval for the treatment of minor health complaints.

Some of the recipes in this book are my at-home versions of classic naturopathic preparations, many of which I learnt how to make in the early days of my degree under the instruction of some incredible herbalists. I distributed the remedies among family, friends and colleagues, and it wasn't long before I was taking orders. Some of them were so popular, in fact, that my own personal stockpile would mysteriously go missing. I use most of the remedies in this book to manage my wellness on a day-to-day basis. From headache to hangover, there's an answer in these pages.

In the next five chapters, you will find a natural remedy that suits your needs at any particular moment.

Note: I'm a big believer in the concept of complementary healthcare, rather than 'alternative medicine'. It's vital that we incorporate natural healthcare measures alongside—as opposed to 'instead of'—the doctor's orders. While herbal medicine is a gentle and safe form of healthcare, I always advise you to check with your GP if you're a little unsure, or if you're already on any medication.

> Some creations are for yummy treats; others are full-blown, palate-blasting tinctures and tonics

## TINCTURES

To make a tincture you'll need a sterilised glass jar (see page 24), your herb or herbs of choice and vodka. (Please see page 58 for alcohol-free alternatives.) The exact amount of vodka required will depend on the density of the herb you're using. For example, dried ginger root is much more dense than something like light and fluffy chamomile flowers. This means that you'll need a lot more vodka to even cover the chamomile than you would the ginger, and you'll end up with a weaker tincture with less concentrated constituents. This is the nature of working with wild materials, so it requires a little understanding of how the strength of a tincture is graded.

We determine the strength of a tincture based on the ratio of dried herb to the amount of liquid, which is called the menstruum and in this instance is vodka. For example, a 1:2 tincture is one part herb to every two parts menstruum. That's 50 grams of herb to every 100 millilitres of vodka. Similarly:

**A 1:3 tincture would be one part herb to three parts vodka (e.g. 200 grams herb and 600 millilitres vodka)**

**A 1:4 tincture would be one part herb to four parts vodka (e.g. 150 grams herb and 600 millilitres vodka)**

Realistically, in a home setting you will only be able to make a tincture of a strength somewhere between 1:4 and 1:8. If you're really lucky, and the starting material is very dense, you might be able to manage a 1:2. Anything more than that really requires professional equipment, or superhuman strength to squeeze the final product out of the herbal material. The recipes in this book all sit between 1:2 and 1:8.

It's also worth noting that if you choose to make your tinctures from fresh herbs rather than dried, they will be less potent due to the concentration of active compounds that occurs during the drying process. So for

It's vital that we incorporate natural healthcare measures alongside—as opposed to 'instead of'—the doctor's orders

example, a 1:2 dried lemon balm tincture, for sleep, will be much stronger acting than a 1:2 fresh lemon balm tincture.

Hopefully I haven't confused you too much, and you haven't run a mile. It's really not that complicated once you get a handle on the idea of tincture strength. As an example though, I'll run you through how to make the basic 1:4 tincture over the page.

# A NOTE ON PRESERVING YOUR REMEDIES

Of course, it's unavoidable that our organic recipes are going to expire before store-bought alternatives, so please take note of the storage suggestions and expiration advice in each one. Always use sterile equipment, and ensure hands and bench tops are squeaky clean. For creams and skin oils, I always add a little vitamin E oil. Not only does it improve skin appearance and elasticity, but it also works to slow the oxidation of the remedies, leaving them fresher for longer. Keep in mind that it won't do anything to prevent microbial growth, so don't be tempted to use any of the remedies in this book beyond the timeframe recommended.

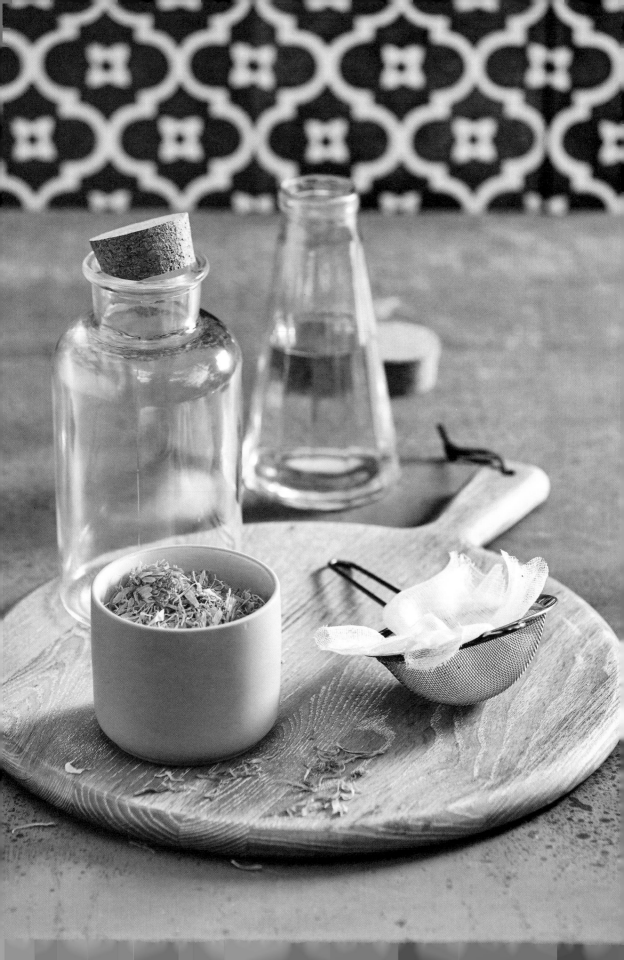

# MAKING A TINCTURE

**1-litre (4-cup) jar (preserving jars are commonly sold in this size)**

**125 g dried herb**

**500 millilitres (2 cups) vodka**

**Step 1**  Grind the dried herb to a powder in a coffee or spice grinder or a mortar and pestle. If you decide to make a fresh plant tincture, you'll need to chop or grate your herbs as finely as possible.

**Step 2**  Place the herbal material in a sterile jar and pour over the vodka. Screw on the lid and shake well to ensure your mix is well combined. Note: if the 500 millilitres doesn't completely cover your herb, then you may need to consider using a larger jar and doubling the amount of vodka. This will result in a 1:8 tincture instead.

**Step 3**  Seal the jar and store it in a cool, dark place for two weeks, making sure you turn it or give it a gentle shake every few days. This ensures the strongest extraction possible.

**Step 4**  Strain the mix through cheesecloth, and discard the solids. You may need to use muscles here and give it a good squeeze to get it all out. Make sure your hands and equipment are nice and clean beforehand, or wear gloves.

**Step 5**  Pour your tincture into a new, sterilised jar and seal. Store in the fridge for up to twelve months.

*Makes 350–400 millilitres of a 1:4 tincture*

It's important to note that you will not end up with 500 millilitres of tincture because your herb will have soaked some up, and it will stubbornly refuse to be squeezed out. It won't affect the strength or efficacy of your remedy, but it will change how much you're left with. A safe assumption is that you'll be left with 20–30 per cent less than how much vodka you use. So this particular recipe will usually give you approximately 350–400 millilitres of tincture. Don't be disheartened if you get less than that, it's just another of the joys of working with natural materials. If you're going to be incorporating your tincture into a more complex remedy, like a cream or a pastille, aim to make more than you think you'll need. It's a much better situation to find yourself in than having too little. And if you have some left over? Well, lucky you!

Depending on your herb and the strength of the extract, doses will sit anywhere between 5 and 30 millilitres. For each of the recipes in this book, I have indicated a safe and effective dose. Not all herbs are dosed at the same level, so I don't recommend you start making tinctures outside of those described in the recipe section of this book unless you are well versed on the topic. Some of my favourite books are listed in the What next? section on page 172 if you want to learn more.

Assuming your vodka is at least 80 proof (40 per cent alcohol), then your tincture could last in the fridge for up to two years, but I would recommend using it up within twelve months and then making a fresh batch. I tend to make a 2–4 week supply at a time, and then have another batch on the go, ready to strain once I've finished my current supply. This is also how the recipes in the

book have been designed. You can, of course, make a larger supply at once, but you'll need a very large jar—or multiple smaller ones—and rather enormous quantities of herbs and vodka.

## A NOTE ON GLYCETRACTS

If you cannot consume alcohol for health, religious or cultural reasons, are avoiding all alcohol before working or driving, or are making a remedy for someone under the legal drinking age, a two-part food-grade vegetable glycerine to one-part water mixture makes a suitable alternative to vodka. Gently heat the water, then stir through the glycerine until completely combined. Pour over the herb in place of vodka. In the Making a Tincture example above, that would equate to approximately 330 millilitres of glycerine and 170 millilitres of water.

Keep in mind that the liquid will be significantly thicker than a tincture and much more difficult to strain through cheesecloth. This may mean you need to water it down slightly just before straining. I would advise adding 500 millilitres (2 cups) water, leaving you with a 1:8 glycetract. If you decide to turn any of the tincture recipes in this book into a glycetract, I advise you to use the methods outlined above to calculate the strength. If you have had to dilute your glycetract prior to straining, you may have to adjust your dose accordingly.

Glycetracts have a shorter shelf life and must be used up within six months of being made. I recommend avoiding both tinctures and glycetracts during pregnancy and while breastfeeding. Instead, stick to infusions and food as medicine.

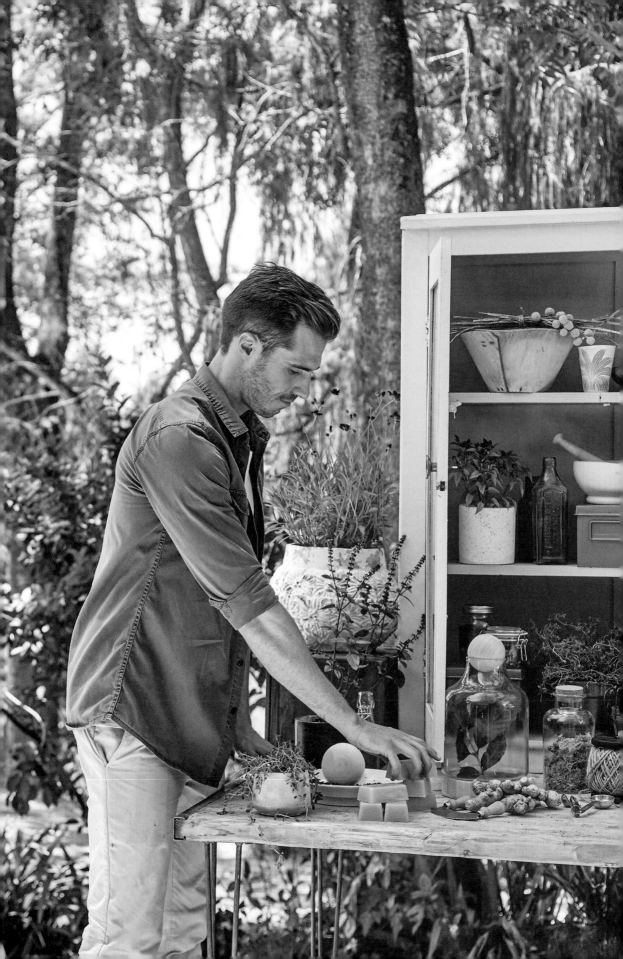

# MAKING AN INFUSED OIL

## YOU WILL NEED

**1 cup dried herbs**

**oil to cover**

## HOW TO

**Step 1** Grind your herb in a coffee or spice grinder. You can't use fresh herbs in oil, so you'll want to dry them first (see page 45) or buy dried herbs to start with.

**Step 2** Place the ground herb into a sterilised jar (see page 24 for how to sterilise a jar), cover with sweet almond oil and leave the sealed jar to rest for two weeks, turning it regularly.

**Step 3** Strain the mix through cheesecloth and transfer to a new sterile jar. Now you've got your oil ready for use, or to incorporate into one of your remedies down the track!

Infused oils should be kept refrigerated and used within six months. As with tinctures, the volume of the end product will be about 20–30 per cent less than the amount of oil you used.

## PREFER COCONUT OIL?

If you like coconut oil more than sweet almond, you'll need to make a hot oil extraction.

**Step 1** Place the oil into a small saucepan and allow it to melt over a very low heat.

**Step 2** Add the ground herbs, stir well and leave on the heat for at least 15–20 minutes, and anywhere up to an hour if you can get the heat low enough.

**Step 3** Allow the oil to cool slightly but not solidify, then strain through a metal strainer lined with cheesecloth. Press with the back of a wooden spoon, as it's burning hot and can't be squeezed by hand. You don't want to be touching it at all while it's hot, and I'd advise wearing gloves just to be safe.

**Step 4** Before it solidifies, pour the infused oil into your sterile jar and leave it to set.

Note: You run the risk of oxidation whenever you bring heat into the equation, so I prefer cold extractions unless you're short on time. Hot oil is also a hazard in the kitchen, so be sure to keep it covered while infusing, ensure it is out of reach of children and exercise care.

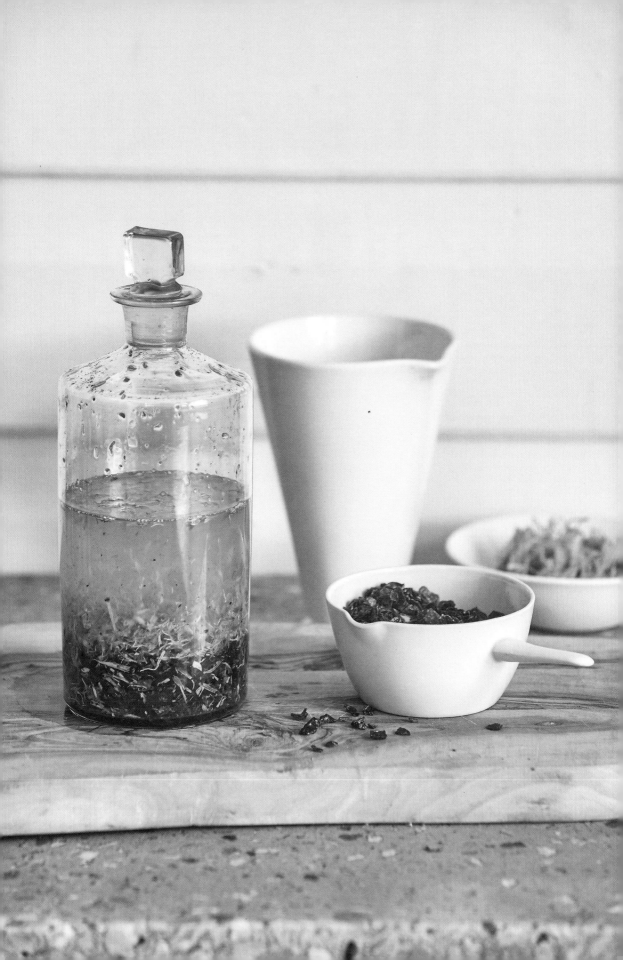

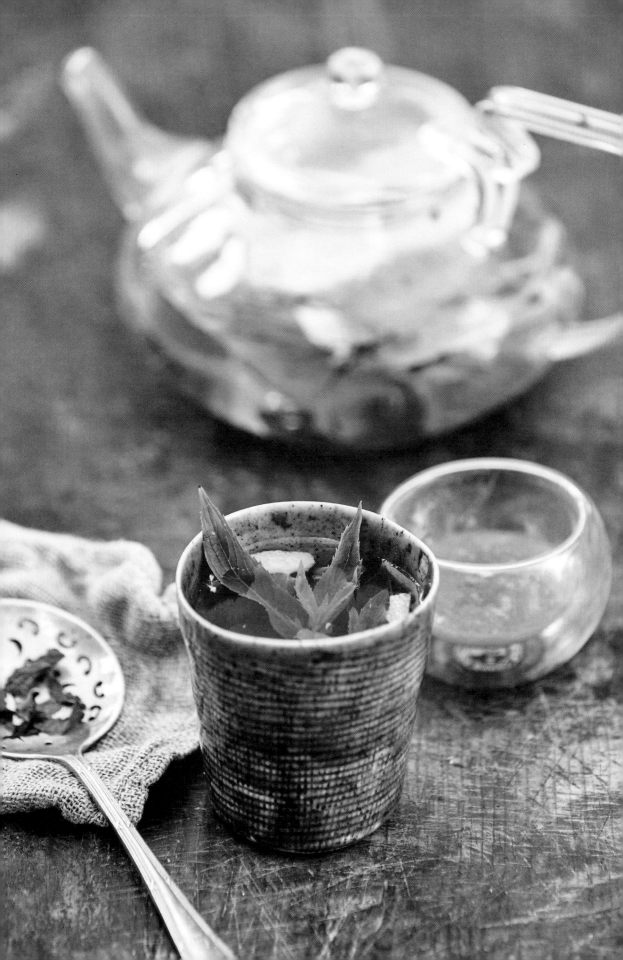

# MAKING AN INFUSION

**1–2 teaspoons of dried herbs or small bunch of fresh herbs**

**boiling water to cover**

## HOW TO

**Step 1** For an infusion, boil the water first and then pour it over the fresh or dried greenery, in a teapot or cup, just like a normal cuppa.

**Step 2** Leave it covered to steep for 8–10 minutes to ensure you get the most out of it, and then strain the water and enjoy.

If you're using herbs with a high oil content—such as lavender or peppermint—make sure you leave a lid on while it brews, or some of the oils will evaporate.

## MAKING A DECOCTION

Forego the electric kettle and use a saucepan and the stovetop instead. We want to draw the goodness from deep within the plant's thick cell walls, and the water needs to be kept boiling to do so.

**Step 1** Place the herb and the water in a saucepan and cover with a lid.

**Step 2** Bring to a boil over a low heat and keep it going for 8–10 minutes. The extra boiling time extracts all the active compounds from the grasp of fibrous shells and husks.

**Step 3** Turn the heat off, strain, and you're ready to go. Teas should be consumed straight away unless you're chilling a big batch in the fridge to enjoy as an iced tea the next day.

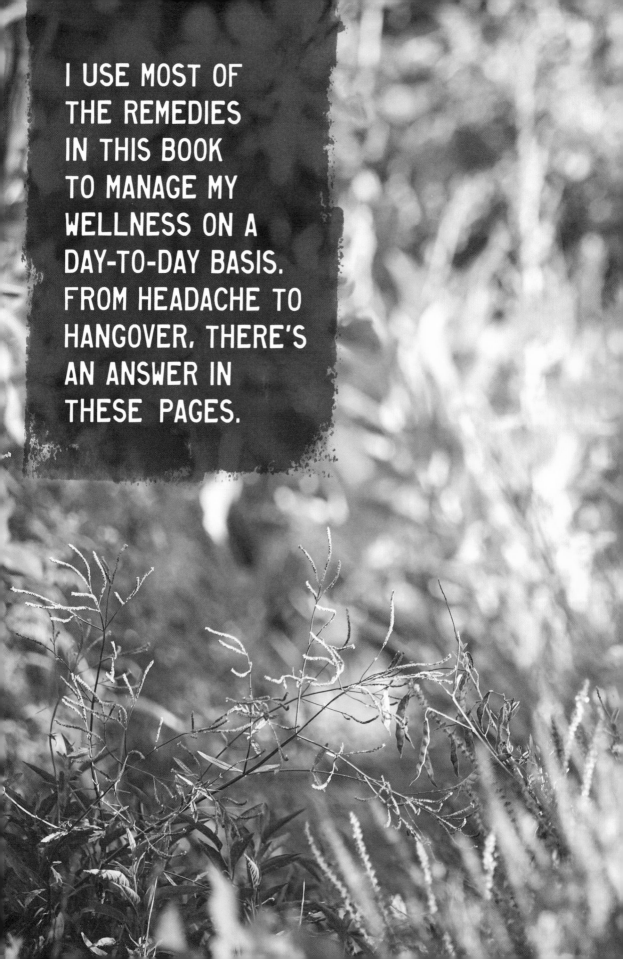

I USE MOST OF THE REMEDIES IN THIS BOOK TO MANAGE MY WELLNESS ON A DAY-TO-DAY BASIS. FROM HEADACHE TO HANGOVER, THERE'S AN ANSWER IN THESE PAGES.

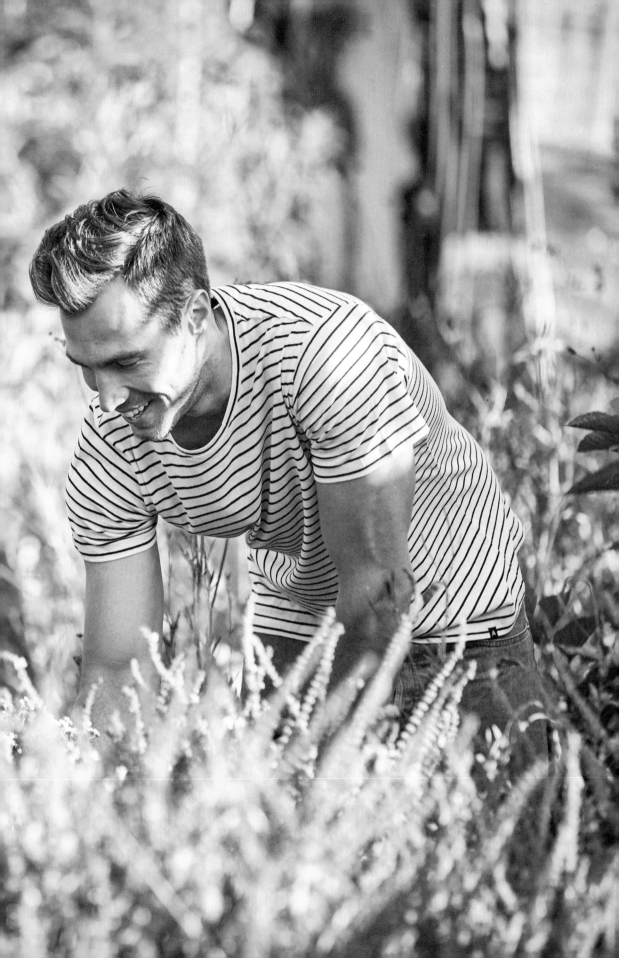

# NATURAL BEAUTY

## Recipes for skin and hair health

**WHEN I STARTED** my web series, it was the natural beauty recipes that received the most overwhelming response. So many awesome herb nerds out there were recreating my recipes for glowing skin and healthy hair, and I realised that I wasn't alone in being aware of the link between beauty and healthy eating. The next logical question then is this: if I've removed certain products from my inside, shouldn't I do it to my outside too? And what can I put *on* my body that will complement everything good that I'm putting *in* it?

The answer is pretty simple: we should put on our bodies, wherever possible, the exact same things that we put in it. Tannins in your morning cup of tea, for example, can counter irritation from shaving; and your bowl of oatmeal can decrease inflammation to leave your skin silky smooth and totally touchable.

So a few years ago, I halved the contents of my bathroom cabinet. I waved goodbye to fragrance-laden moisturisers and cleansers filled with ingredients that I couldn't pronounce, and I headed into the garden. I realised sunburn could be soothed with chamomile, and scratches healed with calendula. Anything that could be made from organic ingredients, I made it.

Of course, I got a few strange looks from housemates when they found my lotions sharing fridge-space with my lunch, but get this: our skin and our digestive tracts are very similar tissues. The gut, of course, is more absorptive, but don't underestimate just how much of what we put on our skin makes its way inside the body. And since it's the largest organ we've got, I'd like to keep my hide healthy.

It's time to get natural with your beauty regime, and this chapter shows you how.

## A NOTE ON BEAUTY REMEDIES

Always test any new remedy on a small patch of skin before using it on larger areas. Even the most natural of ingredients can cause irritation in susceptible individuals. Lavender, aloe vera, and members of the daisy family (such as chamomile and calendula) should be patch tested before they become part of your daily routine.

> We should put on our bodies, wherever possible, the exact same things that we put in it.

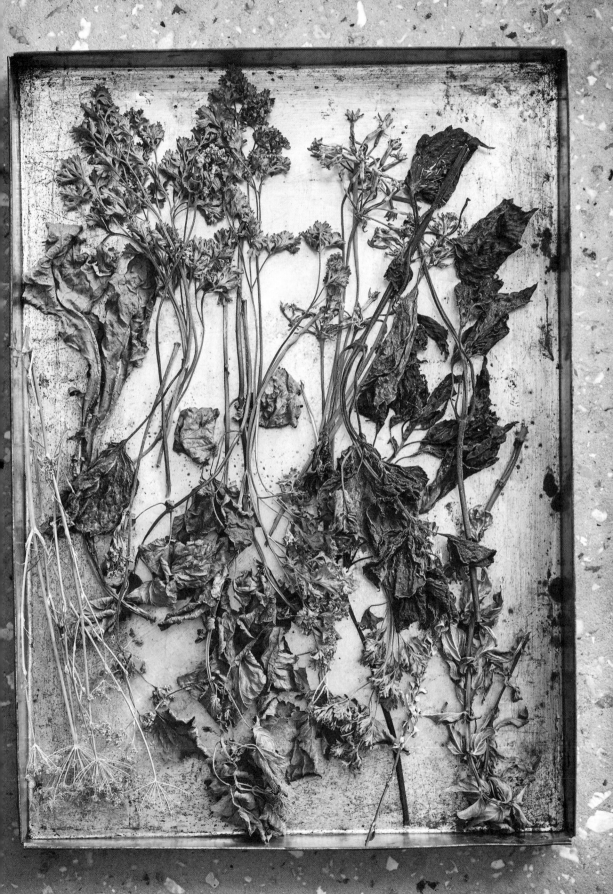

# Skin Repair Body Cream
## —for eczema, cuts and abrasions

If lavender is my favourite calming herb, then calendula would have to be my favourite skin healer. Calendula has a long history as a *vulnerary* herb, meaning that it stimulates tissue repair. We'll start with an infused oil of this bright orange flower, then turn it into a totally clean alternative to commercial body moisturisers, loaded with bonus skin-healing benefits.

## YOU WILL NEED

**3 teaspoons emulsifying wax**

**50 millilitres calendula infused oil (see page 60 for instructions)**

**90 millilitres water**

**10 millilitres calendula tincture (see page 57 for instructions)**

**10–20 drops lavender essential oil**

## HOW TO

**Step 1** Create a double boiler by placing a pyrex bowl over a saucepan with a little water in it. Be careful to make sure that the water doesn't reach the base of the bowl.

**Step 2** Add the emulsifying wax and infused oil to the bowl and bring to a simmer over a low heat. Stir well until all the wax has melted and the two are well combined.

**Step 3** In a second double boiler, combine the water and tincture. Heat the mixture to the same temperature as the wax and infused oil—you'll need a kitchen thermometer to do this!

**Step 4** Slowly (*very* slowly) add the water/tincture mix to the wax/oil, whisking as it cools to maintain the emulsion. If this step is rushed, or if the two components weren't the same temperature to begin with, your cream may split and be ruined.

**Step 5** Transfer to an amber glass jar, and give it an occasional stir until it has cooled and thickened.

**Step 6** Stir through the lavender essential oil.

**Step 7** Seal the jar and transfer to the fridge, to be used within two months.

 **HERB NERD HACK** I also make a chamomile and jasmine version of this cream, which is a much gentler anti-inflammatory and great for those with sensitive skin. Replace the calendula tincture and infused oil with those made from chamomile flowers, and substitute 5-10 drops of jasmine essential oil for the lavender oil.

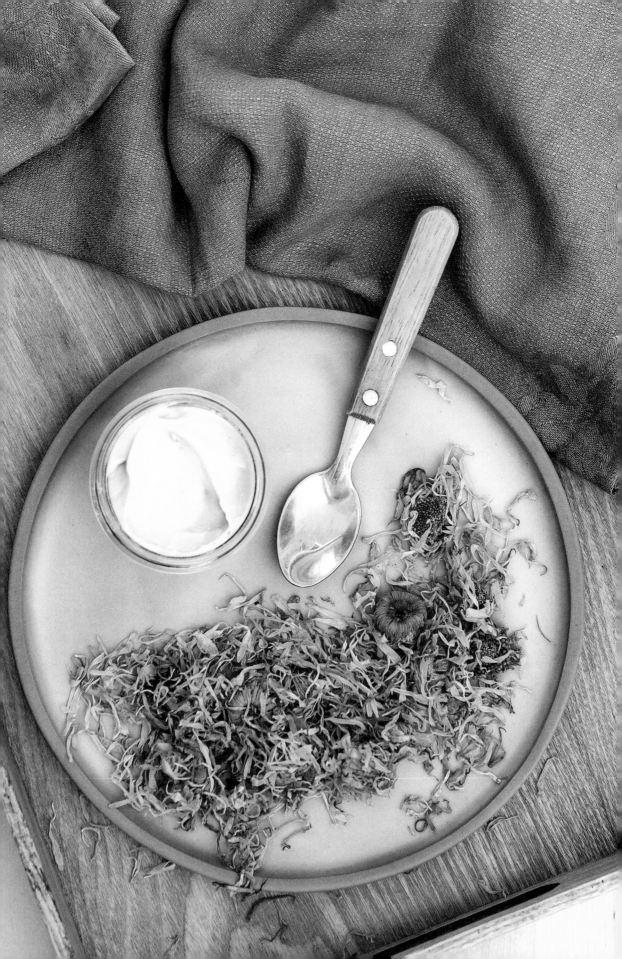

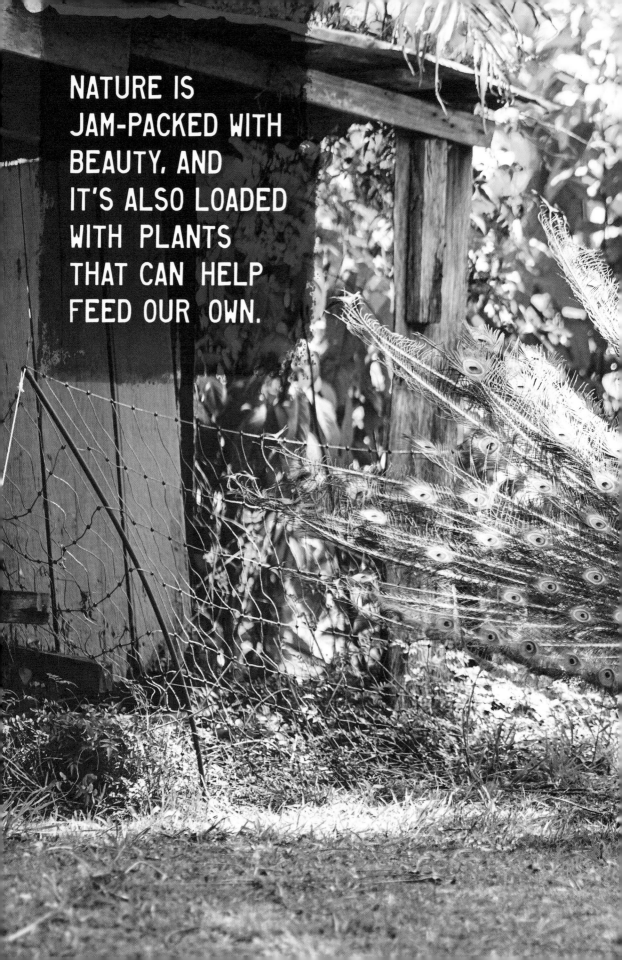

NATURE IS
JAM-PACKED WITH
BEAUTY, AND
IT'S ALSO LOADED
WITH PLANTS
THAT CAN HELP
FEED OUR OWN.

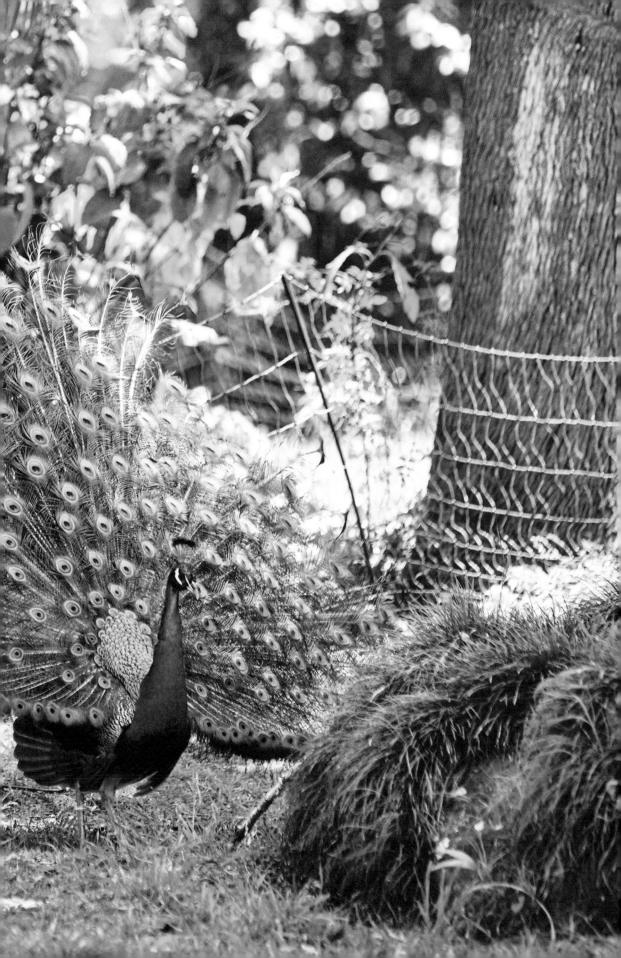

# ALOE EYE GEL

## —for tired eyes

Ditch the slices of cucumber on your eyes; it's all about the homemade eye gel. Supercharged with anti-inflammatory witch hazel—available at most pharmacies—to make that puffiness disappear, this easy-to-make gel hydrates and refreshes. It helps to cover up those sleepless nights, the long-haul travel or the sins of a long weekend.

## YOU WILL NEED

**2–3 large aloe vera leaves**

**5–10 cm length of cucumber**

**1–2 teaspoons witch hazel water**

## HOW TO

**Step 1**  With a sharp knife, slice the top layer of skin away from the aloe vera leaves and scoop out the gel, being careful to get the gel but none of the green fibres. Liquefy the gel in a blender, then pour into a small bowl. Rinse out the blender.

**Step 2**  Roughly chop the cucumber, with the skin on, and place in a blender. Purée, and then strain through cheesecloth. Alternatively, if you have a juicer you can just run it through that. Discard the solids, and pour the juice into a separate bowl.

**Step 3**  With a small fork, whisk together all the aloe gel with some of the cucumber juice and witch hazel water. How much you need of the latter two will depend on the consistency of your gel, but start with one teaspoon of each, and then add a second if there is room without it becoming too watery.

**Step 4**  Store in a sealed glass jar in the fridge for no more than one week, and apply under the eyes as often as required.

 **HERB NERD HACK** In a pinch, black tea bags on their own have a similar *astringent* effect as the witch hazel. Make a cup of tea with two bags, then remove them and allow them to cool to room temperature before placing over your eyes for 10–15 minutes. Don't switch the bags between eyes; it's best to use a clean one on each.

Note: A small number of people with latex allergies will also react to aloe vera, so always test on a small patch of skin before using on your face.

# Lemon Balm Ointment
## —for cold sores

Lemon balm's virus-busting reputation means that if you catch your cold sore in the 'tingle' phase and apply this ointment several times daily, you stand a good chance of reducing its severity. I've also added tea tree oil to this recipe to supercharge its *antimicrobial* (or bacteria-killing) effects.

## YOU WILL NEED

**For the infused oil:**

**30 g dried lemon balm**

**60 millilitres (¼ cup) sweet almond oil**

**For the ointment:**

**12 g beeswax**

**5–10 drops tea tree oil**

## HOW TO

**Step 1** Grind your lemon balm up in a coffee or spice grinder, then place in a sterile glass jar.

**Step 2** Pour over the sweet almond oil, seal the jar and store in a cool, dark place.

**Step 3** After two weeks, strain the mix through cheesecloth. Give it a good squeeze (you may want to wear gloves) and then discard the solids.

**Step 4** Measure out the infused oil. You should have been able to extract around 50 millilitres, but if not you can make up the quantity by adding extra sweet almond oil.

**Step 5** Place a glass bowl over a pot of boiling water to create a double boiler, making sure the base of the bowl doesn't touch the water. Add the infused oil and beeswax, and stir. If your beeswax came in a large block instead of pellets, you'll need to chop it into smaller pieces first.

**Step 6** Once completely melted, pour into a small jar and allow the ointment to cool slightly.

**Step 7** Before it sets, which should only take about 10 minutes, you'll want to stir through the tea tree oil.

**Step 8** Store in the fridge, and apply as needed. Use the ointment within six months.

 **HERB NERD HACK** If you're vegan, replace the beeswax with carnauba wax or cocoa butter.

# ORGANO-OIL
## —for scars and stretch marks

Time is of the essence when it comes to treating scars, and it's best to start this remedy once the wound has sealed shut, but before it develops into a scar; that's when the research suggests it is the most useful. Many people find that it's still worth applying even on old scars and stretch marks though, and there's a reason that the supermarket versions of this remedy fly off the shelves.

## YOU WILL NEED

**1 cup dried calendula petals**

**½ cup dried rose hips**

**1 cup coconut oil**

**½ teaspoon vitamin E oil (optional)**

## HOW TO

**Step 1** Grind the calendula petals and rose hips to a powder in a coffee or spice grinder, then put the powder into a small saucepan.

**Step 2** Add the coconut oil, then place the saucepan over a low heat until the coconut oil has melted, and stir everything together.

**Step 3** Leave over a very low heat for 10 minutes, covered, and then strain through a sieve lined with cheesecloth. Being careful not to get any hot oil on your bare skin, use the back of a wooden spoon to gently squeeze the remaining oil out of the herbs. Discard the solids.

**Step 4** Add the vitamin E oil if you're using it, and stir through.

**Step 5** Pour mixture into an amber glass jar and leave to cool. It will solidify.

**Step 6** Store in the fridge and use within one month, applying to skin two or three times daily. Use liberally on the body, but avoid using the oil on your face.

 **HERB NERD HACK** The added vitamin E increases the shelf life of this preparation and, along with the vitamin C from the rose hips, supports healthy collagen synthesis and skin regeneration. You'll still see good results even if you choose not to include it.

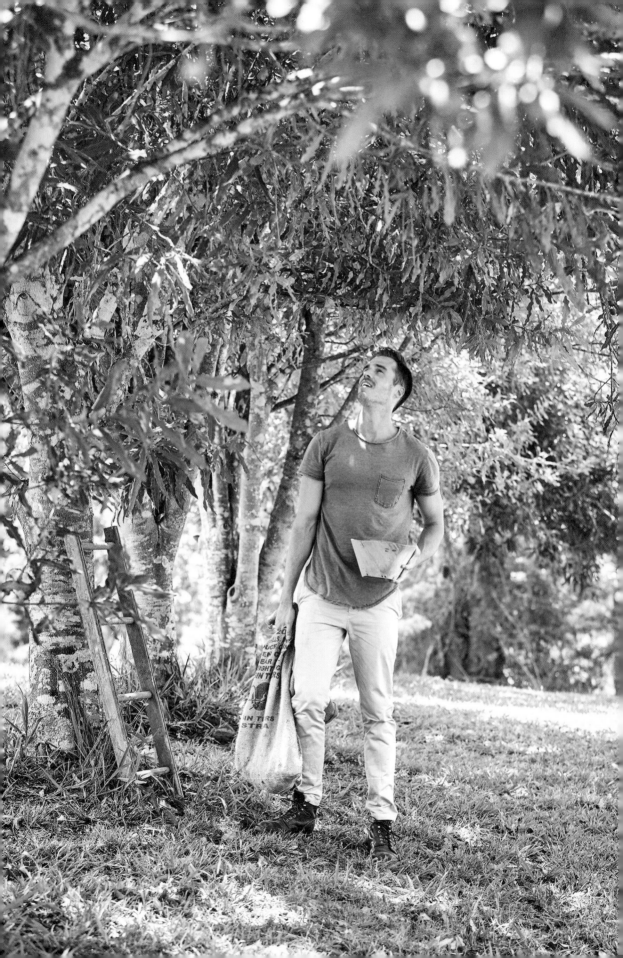

# Kiwi-Berry Face Mask
*— for dry skin*

The fruits in this mask contain alpha-hydroxy acid, an organic compound that helps to exfoliate, making this one great for tired skin. We've also got loads of vitamin C here, which is an essential nutrient for healthy collagen synthesis. As the protein responsible for skin's youthful elasticity, collagen is an important consideration in anti-ageing skincare. Kiwifruit and strawberries also provide a good dose of topical antioxidants to tighten and brighten the skin. Plus, if you get any in your mouth, it tastes so much better than a mask out of a tub!

## YOU WILL NEED

**1 ripe kiwifruit**
**2-3 ripe strawberries**
**Juice of ¼ lime**

## HOW TO

**Step 1** Chop your kiwifruit in half, then scoop out the insides. Discard the skin (or eat it if you'd like—a little extra fibre never hurt!)

**Step 2** Chop the green ends off your strawberries, then mash together with the kiwi flesh.

**Step 3** Squeeze in the lime juice and stir to combine.

**Step 4** Use immediately by applying to the face with a clean brush or your fingers. Avoid the area around the eyes. Leave on for 10-15 minutes, then rinse well with fresh water.

 **HERB NERD HACK** This one is pretty messy! If it's too runny for you, a teaspoon of manuka honey stirred through will give it a little extra stick.

# Honey-Oat Face Mask

*—for oily skin*

This recipe is hugely soothing, and helps absorb excess oils on the skin. Your face will feel clean and soft after rinsing, thanks to the oats.

## YOU WILL NEED

**6 teaspoons whole rolled oats**

**6 teaspoons natural yoghurt**

**1 teaspoon manuka honey**

## HOW TO

**Step 1** Place the oats in a spice grinder and grind to a fine powder, then place in a small mixing bowl or mug.

**Step 2** Add the yoghurt and mix well.

**Step 3** Warm the honey by heating the spoon in a mug of boiled water first (the heat will make it runnier and a little easier to stir through). While still runny, mix the honey through the mask.

**Step 4** This recipe makes one mask and should be used immediately. Apply to clean skin, avoiding the area around the eyes. Leave on for 10–15 minutes, then rinse well with fresh water and a warm, damp cloth.

 **HERB NERD HACK** I choose manuka over regular honey because of its enhanced antibacterial properties. Look for one that has a UMF grade of 15 or higher.

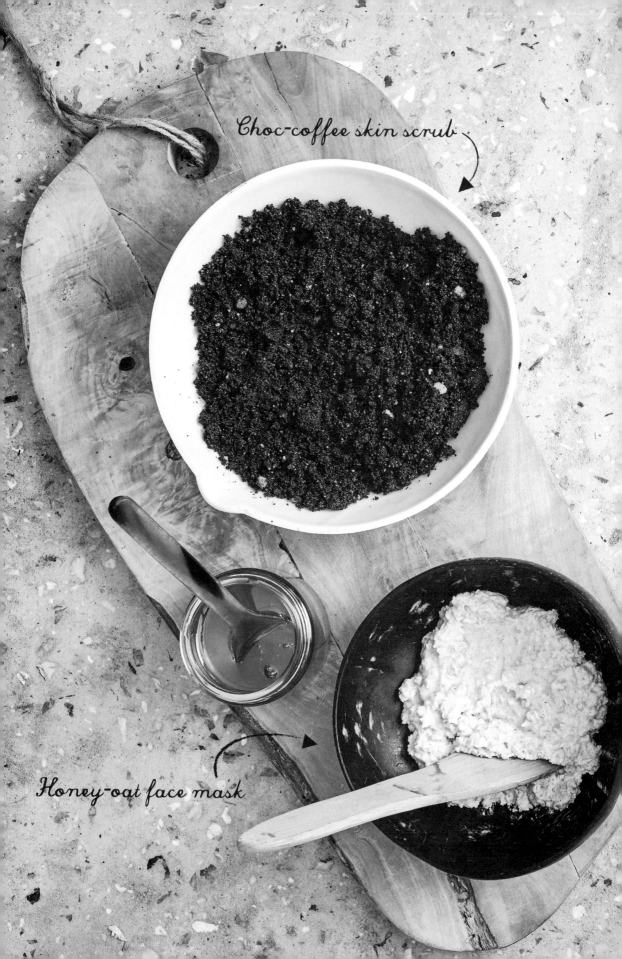

Choc-coffee skin scrub

Honey-oat face mask

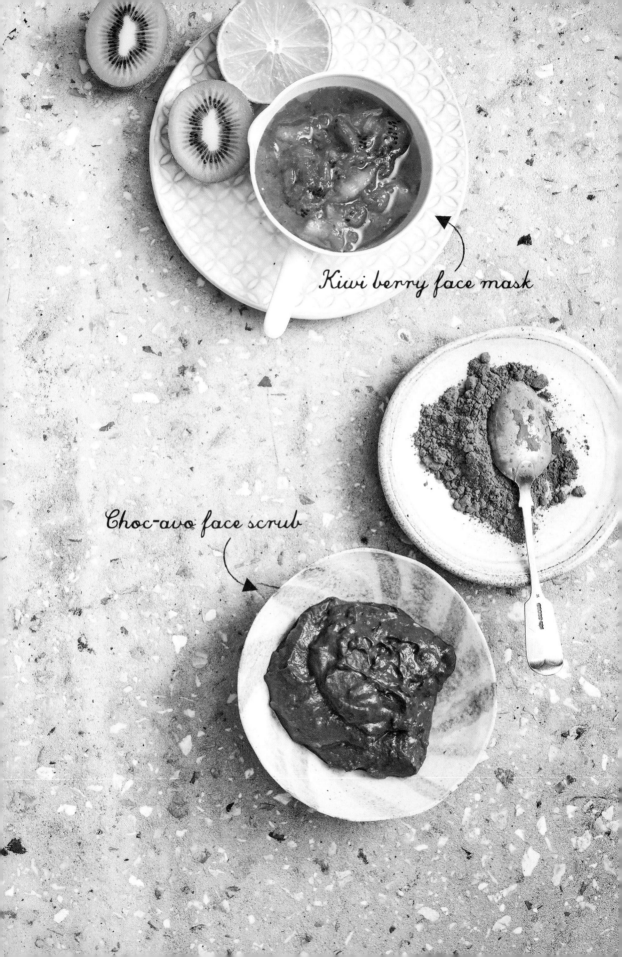

*Kiwi berry face mask*

*Choc-avo face scrub*

# Choc-Avo Face Mask
## —for tired skin

I'm not going to lie, I sometimes put as much of this one in my mouth as I do on my skin. The indulgent combo of avocado and cacao smells just like you're wearing a chocolate cake, and makes this the perfect mask for when you've been neglecting your skin for a while.

## YOU WILL NEED

½ **ripe avocado**

**3 teaspoons raw cacao powder**

**1 teaspoon manuka honey**

## HOW TO

**Step 1** Mash the avocado well, as you don't want any lumpy bits. This is why I err on the side of overripe when it comes to avos!

**Step 2** Stir through the cacao powder until evenly mixed.

**Step 3** Heat a teaspoon in boiling water, then scoop out some honey.

**Step 4** Apply the mask over the face and leave for 10–15 minutes before rinsing off.

 **HERB NERD HACK** Incidentally, with a little coconut cream, vanilla, sea salt and some chia seeds, this recipe becomes a simple chocolate mousse. But hey, why should what we put on our bodies be any different from what we put in them?

# Choc-Coffee Skin Scrub
## —for cellulite

You've seen coffee scrubs popping up everywhere: in health food stores, beauty blogs and—perhaps most of all—on Instagram. It's the caffeine itself that is believed to be behind their cellulite-busting promise, but did you know just how easy these are to make at home? I add a little rosehip oil to the equation to level up on therapeutics.

## YOU WILL NEED

**60 g (¾ cup) ground coffee**

**¼ cup raw cacao**

**9 teaspoons brown sugar**

**18 teaspoons (90 millilitres) sweet almond oil**

**10–20 drops rosehip essential oil**

## HOW TO

**Step 1** Combine the dry ingredients in a bowl and mix well to ensure an even distribution.

**Step 2** Add both of the oils and stir through.

**Step 3** Transfer to a sterile, airtight jar and store in the fridge for up to two weeks.

**Step 4** In the shower, use a small amount of scrub on problem areas, rubbing in a circular motion. Use daily, as best results are seen over time.

 **HERB NERD HACK** Once you've rinsed off, gently pat yourself dry so that you don't completely strip away the moisturising oil and skin-healing rose hip. You'll be left feeling oh-so-soft and smooth!

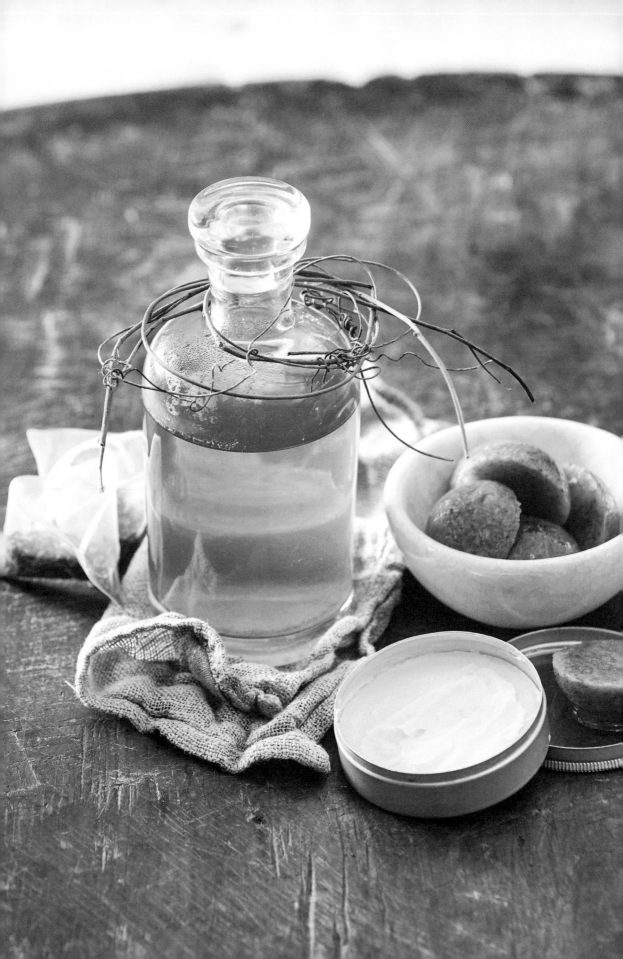

# Green Tea Toner

*—for acne*

I first set foot in a naturopath's office as a pimply teenager. He tweaked my diet, handed me a few supplements to take and advised that I place cool, used green tea bags over my face. 'Weirdo,' I thought at the time; 'genius!' I thought a week later, when I started to see my spots dry up and shrink before my eyes. I've added witch hazel, another *astringent* that you'll find in most pharmacies or large supermarkets; plus lavender essential oil as an antibacterial. I recommend making a fresh batch of this toner each week, and using it twice daily after washing your face.

## YOU WILL NEED

**250 millilitres (1 cup) witch hazel water**

**5 green tea bags**

**5–10 drops lavender essential oil**

## HOW TO

**Step 1** Bring the witch hazel to a boil in a small saucepan over a medium heat.

**Step 2** Turn off the heat, then add the green tea bags and cover with the lid.

**Step 3** Leave to infuse for 10 minutes, then remove the tea bags.

**Step 4** Pour into an amber glass bottle and allow to cool to room temperature.

**Step 5** Once cool, add the essential oil.

**Step 6** Store the bottle in the fridge, and shake well before each use.

**Step 7** To use, soak a few clean cotton wool balls in the toner and wipe over clean skin. If using moisturiser, allow skin to dry first, and use an oil-free moisturiser.

CLOCKWISE FROM LEFT: Green tea toner, Aloe ice, Coconut and peppermint lip balm

# ALOE ICE
## —for sunburn

Prevention is certainly better than cure when it comes to sunburn, but let's face the facts: we Aussies are sun-worshippers. Sometimes, even with the best of intentions, we stay out a little longer than we should and land ourselves an all-too-painful reminder of that hole in the ozone layer. Should you find yourself a little red this summer, you'll be grateful to have a tray of these aloe and calendula ice cubes in the freezer, ready to go. Just pop one out and rub it over the affected area.

They're slippery, stringy little things and will leave calendula petals all over you, but that's part of the goodness. Once you feel like your skin has soaked up as much hydrating gel as it's going to, give the area you are treating a gentle wipe with a cool, damp cloth to clean up the mess. *Makes around 16 cubes that will last three to six months in the freezer.*

## YOU WILL NEED

**6 medium aloe vera leaves**

**1 cup fresh calendula petals, loosely packed**

## HOW TO

**Step 1** Using a sharp knife, remove the top layer of skin from your aloe vera leaves.

**Step 2** With a spoon, scoop out the gel. Remove any green bits; you only want the beautiful clear goo.

**Step 3** Pop the gel in the blender along with the calendula petals and blitz until smooth.

**Step 4** Pour into an ice cube tray—this should fill a standard sized one just about perfectly—and leave in the freezer for at least a couple of hours, until frozen.

 **HERB NERD HACK** Dried calendula will also work in this recipe, as will chamomile flowers from the garden.

Note: As with the eye gel recipe earlier in this chapter, a handful of people may find aloe vera mildly irritating if they have an existing latex allergy. Always patch test before using on sensitive skin.

# PEPPERMINT LIP BALM
## —for chapped lips

This is my homemade version of one of my favourite store-bought lip balms. It is so easy to make in big batches and separate into smaller containers, making great gifts. Alternatively, if you're like me and lose your lip balm every other day, keep them all for yourself!

## YOU WILL NEED

**3 teaspoons coconut oil**

**3 teaspoons shea butter**

**3 teaspoons beeswax pellets (or finely chopped if using a large block)**

**15–20 drops peppermint essential oil**

## HOW TO

**Step 1** In a double boiler, combine the coconut oil, shea butter and beeswax (see page 68 for instructions).

**Step 2** Melt all of the components, stir well and then remove from the heat.

**Step 3** Allow to cool slightly, then stir in the peppermint essential oil.

**Step 4** Transfer to a small glass jar, and apply as necessary to soothe dry or chapped lips.

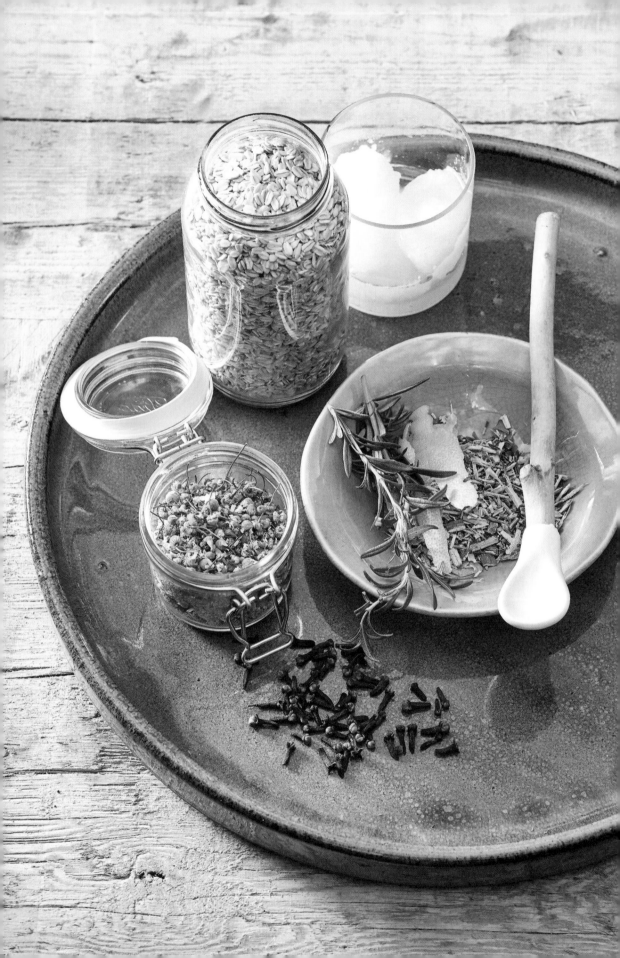

# CLEOPATRA'S BATH MYLK
## —for eczema and dermatitis

There are a few eczema recipes in this book because I get it myself and have had to come up with creative ways to manage it over the years. This is one of my favourites, because for me stress is a real trigger, and this tackles that too. After your bath, you'll be left with skin that feels silky and smooth thanks to the oats. Store the bath mylk in a sealed glass bottle in the fridge, where it will last for about a week. Use it for relief when your skin is particularly irritated, by adding a healthy slurp to a warm bath—the more, the better. It will reduce itchiness and redness, but for real healing, I would follow it up with the skin cream on page 68. Shake well before each use.

## YOU WILL NEED

**500 millilitres (2 cups) coconut milk**

**1 cup fresh or dried chamomile flowers**

**95 g (1 cup) rolled oats**

**500 millilitres (2 cups) boiling water**

**Jasmine essential oil, for fragrance**

## HOW TO

**Step 1** In a heavy-based saucepan, bring the coconut milk to a boil.

**Step 2** Reduce to a simmer, then stir through the chamomile.

**Step 3** After 10 minutes stirring over a very low heat, remove the saucepan from the heat and strain the liquid into a bowl. You may need to press down with a wooden spoon to get all of the liquid out. Discard the solids.

**Step 4** Add the oats to the bowl, combine, then pour over the boiling water. Stir through well, cover and leave to infuse for 5 minutes.

**Step 5** This is where it gets messy! Strain the whole mix through cheesecloth. The oats will have absorbed a lot of the liquid, so you need to squeeze hard to get as much liquid out as you can.

**Step 6** Throw the soggy solids aside, and pour the mylk into a glass bottle.

**Step 7** Allow to cool before adding your essential oil. There is no such thing as too little or too much; this is just for fragrance so the amount you use is up to you and your personal preference.

# Luscious Locks Hair Mask
## —for thin hair

The causes of hair loss are varied, and this is by no means a one-size-fits-all remedy, but for most of us it will help encourage blood flow to the scalp, which carries with it the nutrition necessary to support thick and healthy hair growth. Rosemary is the star attraction here, being a *circulatory stimulant* for the scalp. Regular use is the key here, so make it a weekly ritual to apply this mask for half an hour after washing your hair, then rinse well. Wrapping a towel over your hair will prevent the mask melting all over your face and clothes, and is strongly advised. *Makes enough for one or two applications, depending on hair length.*

## YOU WILL NEED

**½ cup coconut oil**

**20 drops rosemary essential oil**

**10 drops peppermint essential oil**

## HOW TO

**Step 1** Melt the coconut oil over a water bath, then transfer to a shallow, wide container.

**Step 2** Allow to cool somewhat, then stir through the essential oils until well combined.

 **HERB NERD HACK** Ever wondered why rosemary is the herb of remembrance? It's because of its traditional use for increasing blood flow to the brain and improving memory. So you may find that you not only have great hair after using this mask, but that you're a little cleverer too!

# HERBAL MOUTHWASH
## —for oral hygiene

Green tea is *antimicrobial*, killing the bacteria that cause bad breath; cloves are a natural numbing agent; peppermint freshens the breath and leaves you feeling clean. Licorice is a great choice of sweetener because it does so without any cavity-causing sugar. That'll keep your dentist happy!

## YOU WILL NEED

**25 g cloves**

**50 g dried licorice root**

**50 g dried peppermint leaves**

**Peel of one lemon**

**250 millilitres (1 cup) vodka**

**500 millilitres (2 cups) water**

**6 teaspoons green tea leaves (or 5–6 green tea bags)**

## HOW TO

**Step 1** Grind the cloves, licorice and peppermint in a coffee or spice grinder.

**Step 2** Transfer to a sterile glass jar, add the lemon peel and pour over the vodka. Seal, shake well and leave in a cool dark place.

**Step 3** After five to seven days, strain the mix through a sieve lined with cheesecloth, collecting the tincture in a bowl. Use the back of a spoon to press out the extra liquid, or if you're going to squeeze it out, make sure you have very clean hands or are wearing single-use gloves. Discard the solids.

**Step 4** Meanwhile, bring the water to a boil and pour it over the green tea leaves or bags in a glass or ceramic jug. Leave to steep for 10 minutes, then strain. Allow to cool.

**Step 5** Measure out your tincture in a clean measuring jug. Depending on how well you strained it, your efforts should have yielded 150–200 millilitres. Pour in 300–350 millilitres of green tea, to take the volume of mouthwash up to 500 millilitres (2 cups).

**Step 6** Leave to settle, covered, for an hour. Then carefully decant your mouthwash into a fresh sterile jar. Seal and store in the fridge for two to four weeks.

**Step 7** Use after brushing your teeth as usual, by taking a healthy swig, swishing it around your mouth for 60 seconds, then expelling into the sink. Rinse your mouth out again with fresh water to remove any lingering tannins which can stain.

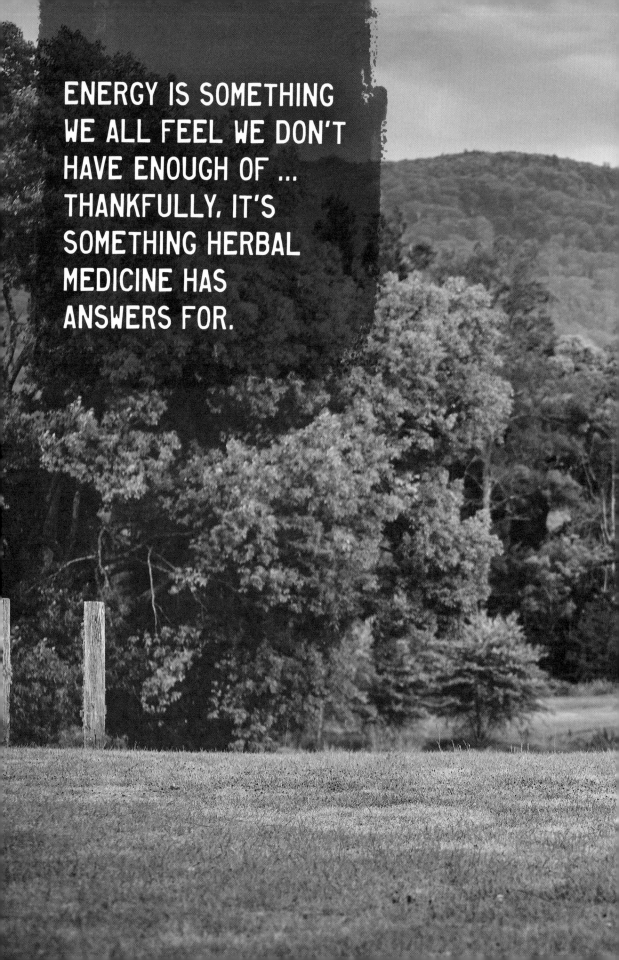

ENERGY IS SOMETHING WE ALL FEEL WE DON'T HAVE ENOUGH OF ... THANKFULLY, IT'S SOMETHING HERBAL MEDICINE HAS ANSWERS FOR.

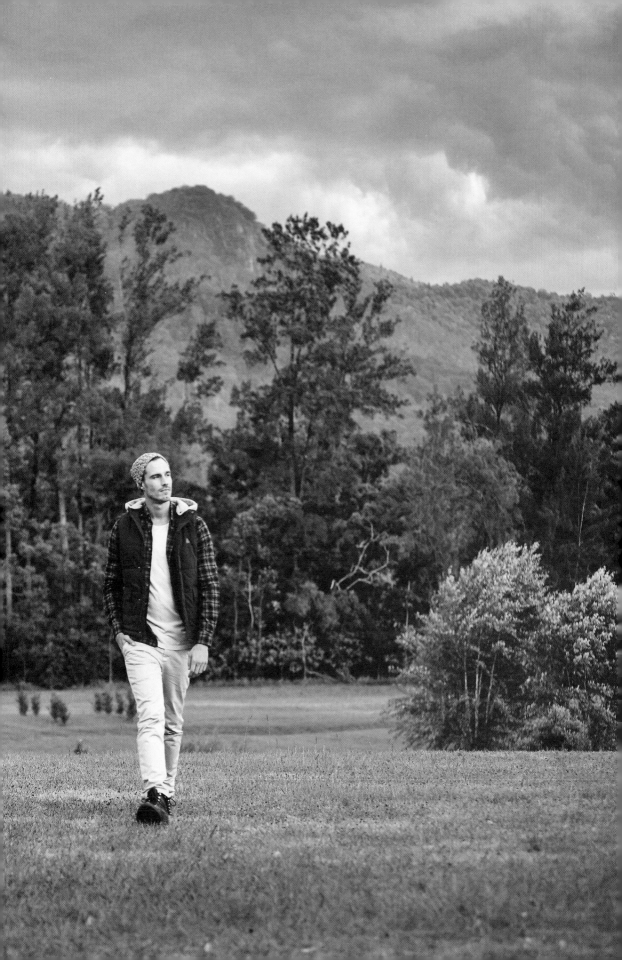

# FOREVER YOUNG

*Remedies to boost energy, mood and libido*

**MY CLINIC SEES** all kinds of presentations, from allergies to autoimmune conditions. Many of these conditions take months—or sometimes years—to get on top of, but other problems can be tackled quickly, so I always ask one question at the end of my first consultation: 'If I can relieve any one complaint for you today, what would it be?' Nine times out of ten, the response is 'I'd really just love to have more energy.'

Energy is something we all feel we don't have enough of, and there are loads of reasons for a decrease in vitality. Thankfully, it's also something that herbal medicine has a lot of answers for.

For me, it was chronic fatigue following a particularly nasty bout of glandular fever—affectionately known as kissing disease—when I was seventeen. I found it tough to recover from the virus, even years after the initial infection had resolved. I felt constantly tired. Every time a cold was going around, you can bet that I got it—and badly! It was actually this experience that led me to see my first naturopath, and have my first taste of herbal medicine.

With a refurbished diet, gradual exercise and loads of herbal *adaptogens*, I recovered. Adaptogens, in case you were wondering, are herbs that were traditionally used to improve a person's resistance to external stressors. They are a varied group in terms of how they work, but an invaluable tool for any herbalist. Alongside herbs to nurture my nervous and immune systems, they helped bring me back to full health.

And the kiss was totally worth it, in case you were wondering. These days, however, I have a new energy-vampire to contend with. It's one that we're all familiar with: stress.

Stress on its own isn't a bad thing, and was an essential evolutionary step so that we had the 'get up and go' to hunt for food and

> Adaptogens are herbs that were traditionally used to improve a person's resistance to external stressors.

run away from sabre-tooth tigers. These days though, there are fewer sabre-tooth tigers around, and yet we're probably relying on our stress response more heavily than ever. We use it to be efficient at work, flooding our veins with caffeine and sugar to keep us going even when our bodies are crying for us to stop. Caffeine blocks the adenosine receptors in our bodies, which in turn keeps us awake and alert. We squeeze out every ounce of adrenaline and cortisol that we can, in an attempt to fit more hours into our days. Even our weekends lose their status as rest days, as we try and run all the errands we couldn't get done during the week.

And so begins the cycle of premature ageing. We can't sleep because we bring work stress into our beds; we wake up looking and feeling tired; we continue the cycle with a triple-shot latte in the morning. Immunity, digestion, mood, libido and appearance all take a hit when the stress monster comes out. Exercise is important, and there are remedies that can help support it. Working out is best done in the morning, as it respects your natural hormonal rhythm. It gets your body and mind going first thing in the morning, when cortisol should be at its highest, then leaves the evening for wind down time so that melatonin can do its work and put you to sleep. I've always been a morning exerciser, but I also used to be guilty of using store-bought pre-workout powders to amplify my sweat sessions. They are full of stimulants and always left me feeling rubbish afterwards.

So I set out to make my own cleaner version, and stumbled upon matcha. Matcha is a bit of a favourite of mine, as it has all the goodness of green tea but better, because you are quite literally ingesting the whole leaf ground up. See the Matcha Warrior recipe on page 96.

> We can't sleep because we bring work stress into our beds; we wake up looking and feeling tired; we continue the cycle with a triple-shot latte in the morning.

Another unfortunate side effect of chronic stress and depleted vitality is a drop in libido. For that, I have created a cheeky herbal shot on page 97. When I posted the first incarnation of this recipe online, it was only hours before I got an email asking whether or not it was safe to slip into a husband's drink to give him a little more 'oomph'. Apart from the fact that she'd never have gotten away with it (damiana leaves a tell-tale herbaceous flavour that cuts right through the cherry), I definitely don't recommend trying to give your partner a shot of this without them knowing. This remedy packs a punch. I've had a few couples, especially the other side of middle age, who have told me that the Korean ginseng works wonders for them.

It's important to note that for long-term wellness, it's essential to work on stress management, to strive for a healthy work–life balance and to ensure we are nourishing our bodies with all of the micronutrients to support ourselves through short bursts of *necessary* stress. However, if you need a little herbal help along the way, the following recipes might be just the thing.

# OVERNIGHT OATS
## —to safeguard from stress

The humble oat might seem like an unlikely herbal hero at first sight, but *Avena sativa* is actually one of the best *nervine* herbs, which is a class of ingredients traditionally believed to support healthy nervous system function. They're the perfect way to get your day off to a good start! Why go to the effort of making a tincture when they make such a simple (and delicious) breakfast.

Overnight oats require less work than porridge, and are more suitable to our warm Aussie climate. I make mine up in jars so that they are waiting for me in the morning; they're the perfect on-the-go brekkie!

## YOU WILL NEED

**75 g (¾ cup) whole rolled oats**

**130 g (½ cup) natural yoghurt, or a dairy-free substitute like coconut yoghurt**

**125 millilitres (½ cup) almond milk**

**1 teaspoon rice malt syrup, honey or a pinch of stevia (optional)**

## HOW TO

**Step 1** Mix all of the ingredients together in a bowl, then transfer to a jar or glass container. Seal, and leave in the fridge overnight.

**Step 2** In the morning, the oats can be topped with your favourite fruits, nuts and seeds, or use one of my favourite combos below!

### ROSEWATER AND PISTACHIO

Stir through a teaspoon of rosewater and a pinch of ground cardamom, then top with one or two tablespoons of crushed raw pistachios to serve.

### POMEGRANATE AND CACAO NIB

Add ¼ cup pomegranate seeds or flesh to the mix before leaving it overnight, then sprinkle a teaspoon of raw cacao nibs over the top to serve.

### LIME AND COCONUT

Before leaving to soak overnight, add the grated zest of one lime, as well as half of its juice. The next morning, sprinkle a tablespoon of toasted coconut flakes over the top to serve.

 **HERB NERD HACK** Oats are also an incredible ally in the battle against bad cholesterol. They contain fibres called beta-glucans that bind and remove cholesterol from the body, improving blood lipid levels.

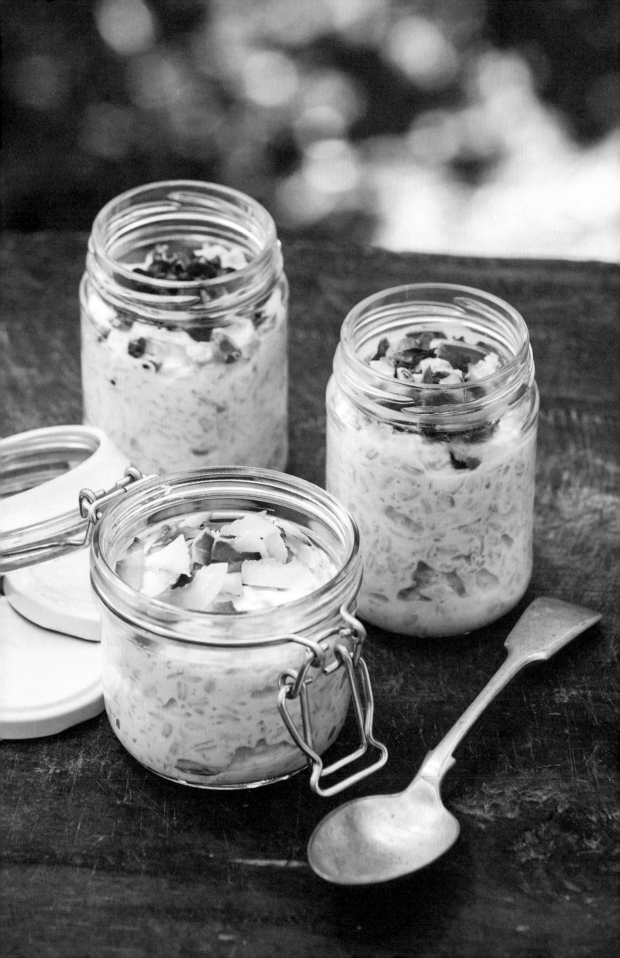

# Matcha Warrior

## —a pre-workout powder

Green tea has been linked to a whole host of benefits because of its xanthines and catechins. You don't need to remember these funny words, all you need to know is that matcha is an amazing metabolism booster. A pinch of cayenne warms the body up, and lemon gets digestion going for the morning. Don't expect the 'zing' you would get from a store-bought alternative, but I bet you'll find this makes you sweat like nothing else.

Up until now it's been my little fitness secret, but I guess the secret's out!

## YOU WILL NEED

¼ cup matcha green tea powder

3 teaspoons lemon juice powder

Pinch of cayenne pepper

Pinch of stevia (optional, but I prefer mine without)

## HOW TO

**Step 1** Combine all the ingredients together in a small bowl, and then store in an airtight container. Due to the organic nature of this product, it may clump in time. To avoid this happening, keep it well sealed and in a dry place.

**Step 2** To use, add up to a teaspoon of the powder to a gym shaker with a few blocks of ice (it tastes best cold). Add water, and shake well.

**Step 3** Now go move that body!

Note: As with any source of caffeine, caution is advised if you're prone to high blood pressure. If in doubt, check with your doctor before using this remedy.

# LIBIDO-BOOST SHOT
## —aphrodisiac

Although these herbs are safe and effective in both sexes, it's men who will likely see the biggest benefit. They're a bit more exotic than some other ingredients we've used so far, but I think you'll find it's well worth your time to hunt them down.

## YOU WILL NEED

**25 g dried damiana leaves**

**25 g dried Korean ginseng**

**Peel of one orange**

**200 millilitres vodka**

**300 millilitres cherry concentrate**

## HOW TO

**Step 1** Grind the damiana and ginseng into a powder with a mortar and pestle, or a coffee or spice grinder. Combine the two in a large, sterile jar.

**Step 2** Add the orange peel and cover with the vodka.

**Step 3** Leave for five to seven days in a dark place, giving the jar a shake each day.

**Step 4** Pour in the cherry concentrate, replace the lid and shake well, being sure to get all of the herb away from the side of the jar.

**Step 5** Strain and discard the solids.

**Step 6** Pour the liquid into a sterilised bottle. You may find that over an hour or two, a sediment forms on the bottom. That's just leftover herb, so feel free to decant the liquid off the top.

**Step 7** Enjoy one or two 30 millilitre shots, and whatever follows. Because we've diluted the alcohol, I recommend you store it in the fridge and use it within two to four weeks of making.

 **HERB NERD HACK** A little of this is a good thing, but too much and you may find the excess alcohol having the opposite effect!

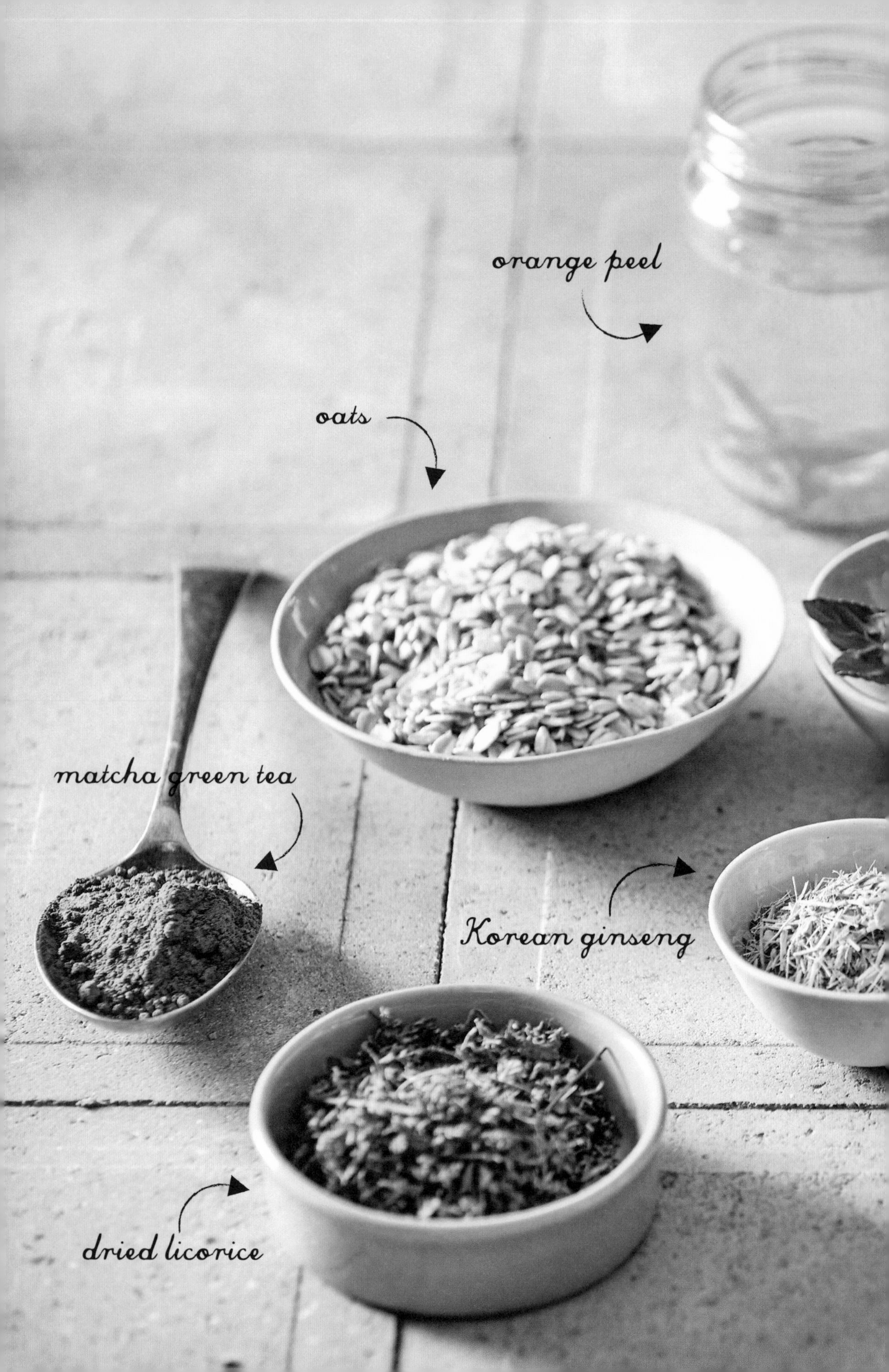

orange peel

oats

matcha green tea

Korean ginseng

dried licorice

vodka

dried chamomile

brahmi

dried rose petals

# HANGOVER SHERBET
## —for the morning after

Ideally, you won't need this (it's really best to limit your alcohol intake), but if you do happen to slip up, here's a little herbal hack that will help your recovery. I'm going to be upfront with you on this one: don't expect it to be a sugary treat. Rather than the candy aisle, I took my inspiration from old first aid rehydration salts, then removed the refined sugar and replaced it with softly sweet pineapple and raspberry. Avoid powdered juices and opt for the freeze-dried whole fruit instead, as it'll keep the sugar load down. Remember though that the main aim of this remedy is to deliver a therapeutic dose of ginger to settle your nausea, so keep in mind that the end product packs a spicy punch.

Although there's no herb in here to directly treat the headache component of a hangover, taking three teaspoons of this in at least 500 millilitres (2 cups) of water once or twice in the day will help rehydrate you, deliver vital electrolytes and speed up your recovery. This recipe will give you a big supply, and it will keep for three to four months if stored in a sealed jar away from any moisture.

## YOU WILL NEED

½ **cup pineapple powder**
¼ **cup raspberry powder**
¼ **cup dried ginger, ground**
¼ **cup citric acid**
¼ **cup bicarbonate of soda**
½ **teaspoon sea salt**

## HOW TO

**Step 1** In a medium-sized bowl, combine all of the powders thoroughly.

**Step 2** Grind the sea salt between your fingers and thumb to make sure the particles are small, then stir through the sherbet until evenly dispersed.

**Step 3** Transfer to a sterilised, very dry jar. Enjoy three teaspoons in a large glass of water.

 **HERB NERD HACK** If you are prone to acid reflux, this remedy may not be for you. Alcohol consumption increases stomach acid and can be wearing on the lining, so citric acid might aggravate your condition. Consider decreasing the quantity of citric acid or removing it completely, but keep in mind that you'll lose the fizz factor and the flavour will take a bit of an unpleasant turn.

# 'Pep Me Up' Peppermint Mist
## —for mental clarity

A bottle of this should always be sitting on your desk, ready to spritz when the dreaded 3 pm brain fog hits. Peppermint oil is used in aromatherapy to invigorate the mind and increase alertness. I used to rely on it to keep me on track during exam time, when my brain was already slipping into holiday mode and stubbornly refusing to hold on to new information. This is a more sophisticated version of my study remedy, with added glycerine and rose petals, so that you know you're doing something good for your skin at the same time.

## YOU WILL NEED

**2 red or deep pink roses**

**250 millilitres (1 cup) boiling water**

**6 teaspoons vegetable glycerine**

**20 drops peppermint essential oil**

## HOW TO

**Step 1** Make an infusion by tearing off the rose petals, placing them in a bowl and pouring over the boiling water. Cover, and leave to rest for 10 minutes before straining. Discard the petals.

**Step 2** Stir through the vegetable glycerine, then leave to cool.

**Step 3** Pour into a spray bottle, then add the essential oil. Replace the lid and shake well.

**Step 4** Lightly spritz your face as often as required, or spray into the air to enjoy its aromatherapy benefits. This batch will last up to a month if kept in a cool place.

 **HERB NERD HACK** Wild rose varieties are best for this remedy, but any red or deep pink roses will do at a pinch. Use what you've got growing in your garden if you can!

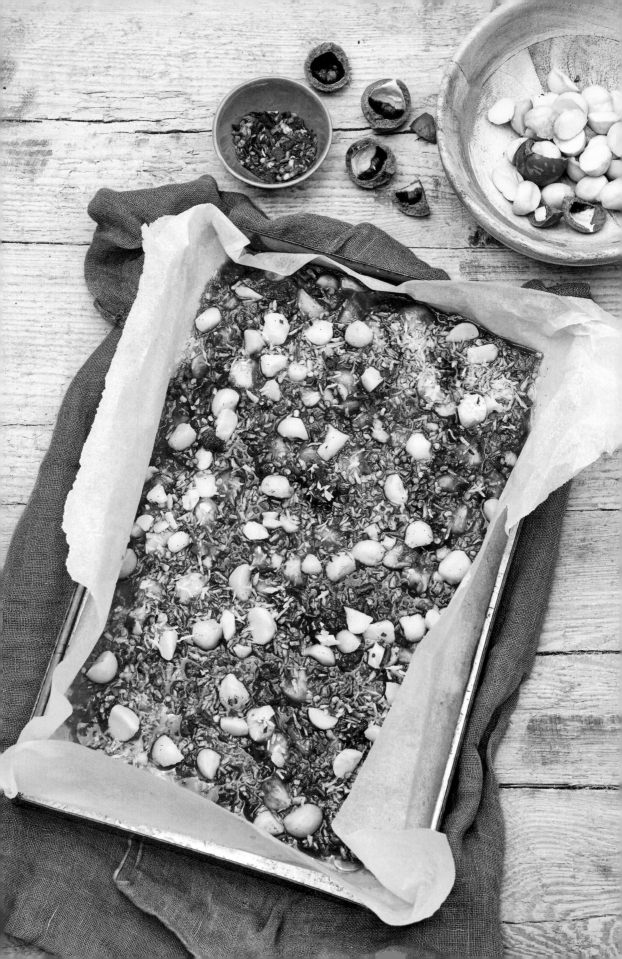

# MACA-MACADAMIA CHOCOLATE BARK

*—to bust a bad mood*

I know what you're thinking: chocolate will lift anyone's mood. And it's true! But I've taken the mood-altering powers of raw cacao, and removed any trace of dairy or refined sugars. I've also added powdered maca root, an Incan *adaptogen* that was once reserved for their best warriors. Wearied warrior or not, this low-fructose treat can be enjoyed in moderation on those days when you feel like a little pick-me-up. *Makes twelve serves.*

## YOU WILL NEED

**1 vanilla bean pod**

**155 g (1 cup) macadamia nuts**

**½ cup coconut oil**

**125 g (½ cup) coconut cream**

**¼ cup raw cacao powder**

**9 teaspoons dried maca root powder**

**9 teaspoons (45 millilitres) rice malt syrup**

**Pinch of sea salt**

**¼ teaspoon dried chilli powder**

**¼ cup shredded coconut**

## HOW TO

**Step 1** Slice the vanilla pod lengthways, then scrape out the seeds using the back of a knife. Discard the pod and keep the seeds.

**Step 2** Roughly chop the macadamias in half, and place to one side for later.

**Step 3** Melt the coconut oil in a large mixing bowl over a water bath.

**Step 4** Remove bowl from heat and stir through the coconut cream, cacao, vanilla seeds, maca, rice malt syrup, sea salt and chilli powder. Whisk until smooth.

**Step 5** Add half the macadamias and half the coconut. Stir through with a wooden spoon or spatula.

**Step 6** Line a baking tray with baking paper, then spread the mixture over evenly.

**Step 7** Top with the remaining macadamias and coconut.

**Step 8** Refrigerate until set, then break into twelve pieces roughly the same size. To store, layer the pieces in an airtight container, separated by baking paper. Keep refrigerated or—if like me you prefer it with a little more snap to it—in the freezer.

# 'FORGET-ME-NOT' SALSA VERDE
## —for better memory

In Ayurveda, gotu kola is what's known as a *rasayana* (rejuvenating) remedy, said to improve memory and prolong lifespan. I was lucky enough that my mates, the lovely Ratnayake family, introduced me to Bandu, who has a garden overflowing with the stuff. He generously gave me enough to make bucket loads of this recipe.

I serve this herbaceous sauce over fresh grilled prawns, but it tastes just as great on meats, fish or roast veggies. You need to have a small amount every day to reap the rewards. *Serves 4 as an appetiser.*

## YOU WILL NEED

### Salsa

**1 cup fresh gotu kola leaves, loosely packed**

**1 cup fresh basil leaves, loosely packed**

**1 cup fresh flat-leaf parsley, loosely packed**

**2 garlic cloves, crushed**

**3 teaspoons capers**

**1 anchovy fillet, roughly chopped**

**2 bird's eye chillis, seeds removed**

**90 millilitres olive oil**

**Juice of 1 lemon**

**Sea salt and freshly ground black pepper, to taste**

### Prawns

**16 king prawns, shelled and deveined**

**3 teaspoons olive oil**

**Pinch each of sea salt and freshly ground black pepper.**

## HOW TO

### Salsa

**Step 1** Wash your herbs thoroughly and dry in a salad spinner, or leave to dry on absorbent paper for a few hours.

**Step 2** Place all the ingredients in a blender and blitz until smooth.

**Step 3** Store in the fridge in a sealed container, and use within the week.

## HOW DO I USE IT?

### Prawns

**Step 1** Place the prawns in a bowl and stir to coat with the oil, salt and pepper. Cover with plastic wrap, and leave the prawns at room temperature for at least 15 minutes.

**Step 2** Meanwhile, heat the barbecue or place a grill plate over a high heat. You need to cook the prawns on a very hot surface.

**Step 3** Without any extra oil, cook the prawns for a minute on each side.

**Step 4** Arrange on a plate and cover with foil for 2–3 minutes before serving.

**Step 5** Serve with a generous dollop of the salsa verde to enjoy the memory-boosting effects of gotu kola!

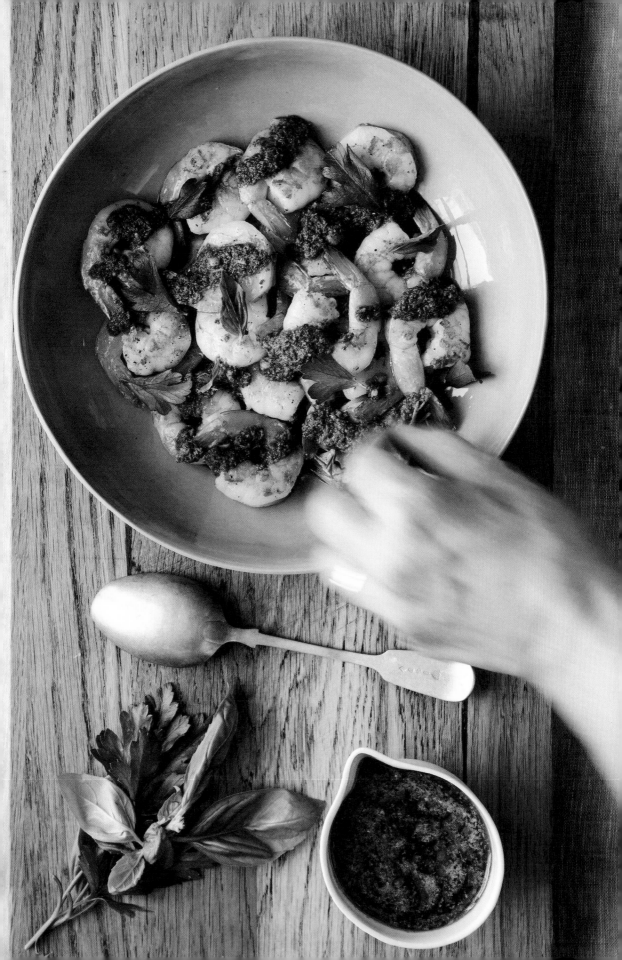

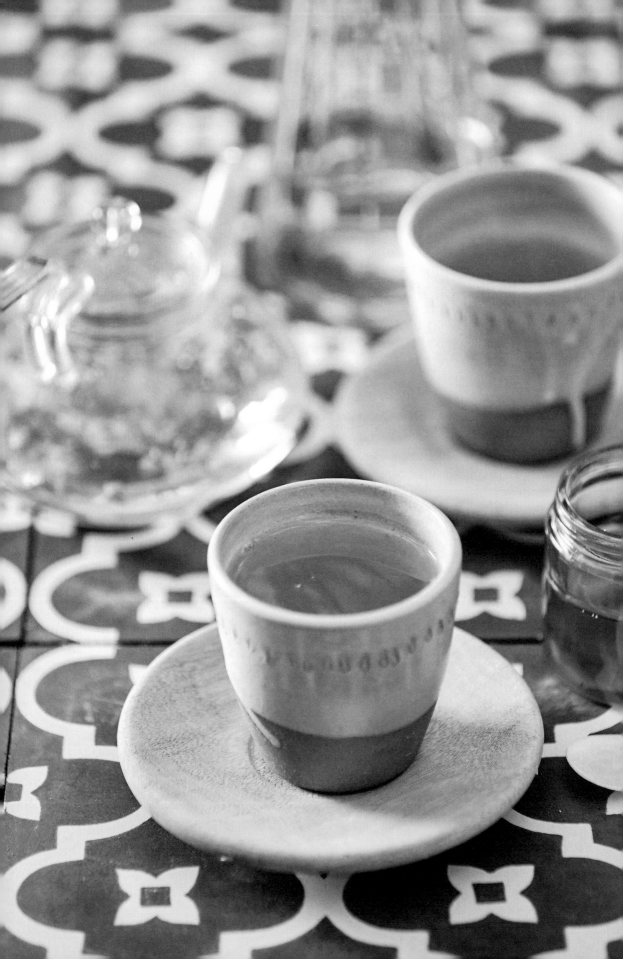

# Fresh Feverfew Tea
## —for migraines

I have a friend who gets debilitating migraines, and I have witnessed first-hand just how awful they can be. There's no herb strong enough to beat one down once it's kicked in, but feverfew can be used as a preventative measure. If you are prone to painful migraines, consider growing this in your garden, and brew an infusion every day. You'll want to make sure you get the correct species, *Tanacetum parthenium*, which has small white and yellow flowers that look like little daisies.

## YOU WILL NEED

**1–2 tablespoons fresh feverfew leaves, chopped**

**250 millilitres (1 cup) boiling water**

**Stevia, to taste**

## HOW TO

**Step 1** Place the leaves in a mug and pour over the boiling water. Cover, and leave to steep for 8–10 minutes.

**Step 2** Taste, and add stevia as necessary. Feverfew on its own is quite bitter, but so much better than a migraine!

 **HERB NERD HACK** If tension headaches are more of a concern for you than migraines, the remedy couldn't be simpler: a drop of peppermint essential oil rubbed onto each temple has been compared to a standard dose of paracetamol—easy!

# JOY-IN-A-JAR TINCTURE
## —to improve your mood

The verdict is in: St John's Wort is without a doubt one of nature's most effective offerings for improving mood. I've combined it with other *thymoleptic* herbs, which positively enhance your mood, to create something that I think feels like a hug in a bottle.

## YOU WILL NEED

**Large bunch fresh lemon balm, finely chopped**

**8–10 fresh lavender heads**

**125 g dried St John's Wort**

**500 millilitres (2 cups) vodka**

## HOW TO

**Step 1**  Wash the fresh herbs well, then leave them to dry on absorbent paper.

**Step 2**  Grind the St John's Wort to a powder using a coffee or spice grinder.

**Step 3**  Pack the fresh lavender, lemon balm and St John's Wort powder into a glass jar, then cover with vodka.

**Step 4**  Replace the lid, and shake well to ensure the contents are well mixed.

**Step 5**  Place the jar in a cool, dark place for two weeks. Shake the jar gently every day to keep the herbs from settling.

**Step 6**  After two weeks, strain the mixture through cheesecloth and discard the solids. Pour the tincture into a sterilised jar.

**Step 7**  Start with one teaspoon daily, in a little water, or grape juice if you want to mask the flavour of your medicine. You can bump it up to two if you feel the need, but definitely no more than that. This remedy works best with daily use, and you should feel real change happen between two to six weeks.

Note: Always consult your doctor before taking St John's Wort in any form. St John's Wort can increase or decrease the effects of other drugs and should not be taken in combination with any other medication or prescription—especially antidepressants or the contraceptive pill.

If you prefer to make an alcohol-free version of this remedy, please use the glycetract method (see page 58).

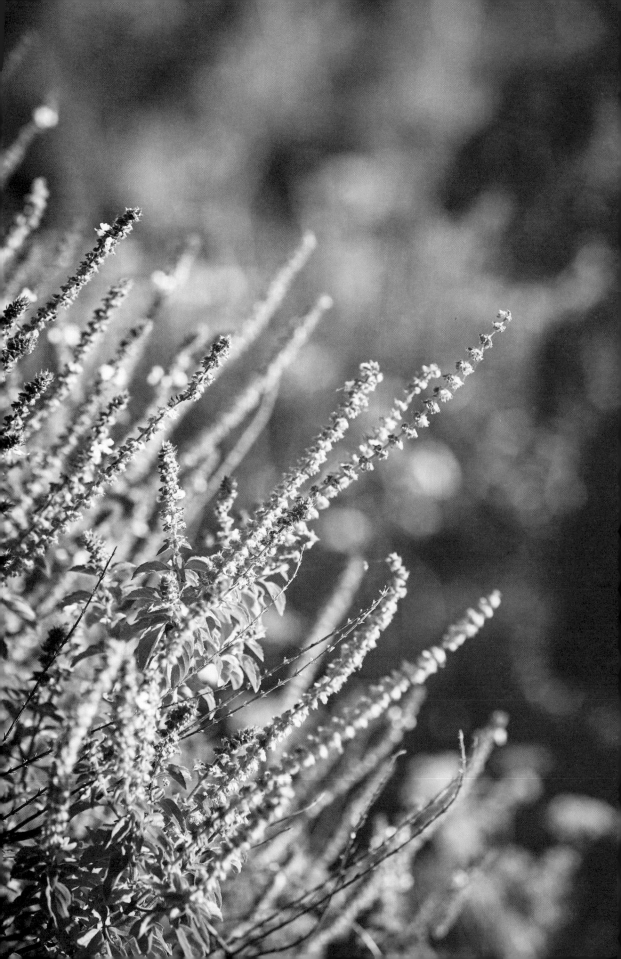

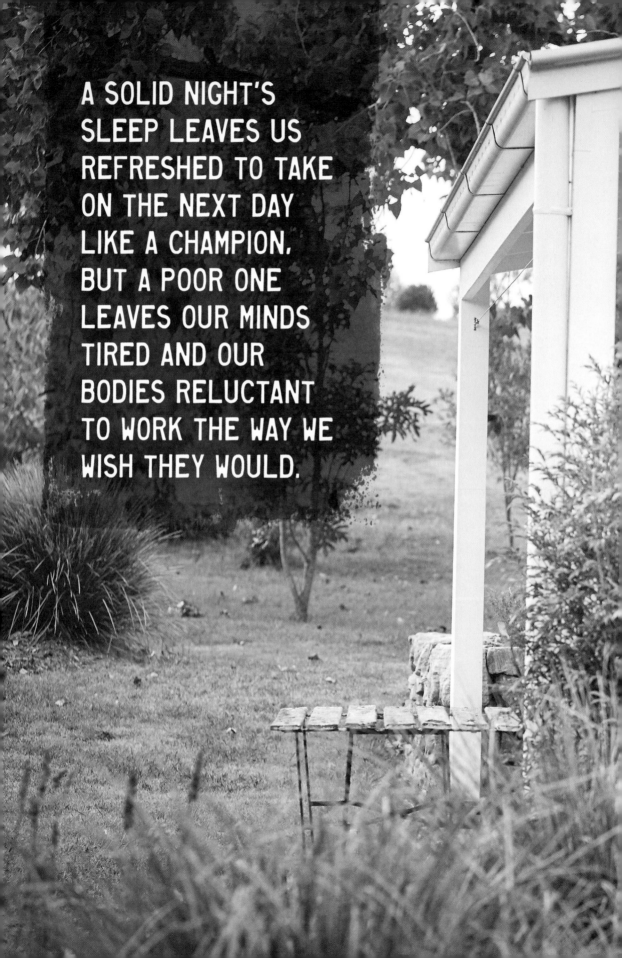

A SOLID NIGHT'S SLEEP LEAVES US REFRESHED TO TAKE ON THE NEXT DAY LIKE A CHAMPION, BUT A POOR ONE LEAVES OUR MINDS TIRED AND OUR BODIES RELUCTANT TO WORK THE WAY WE WISH THEY WOULD.

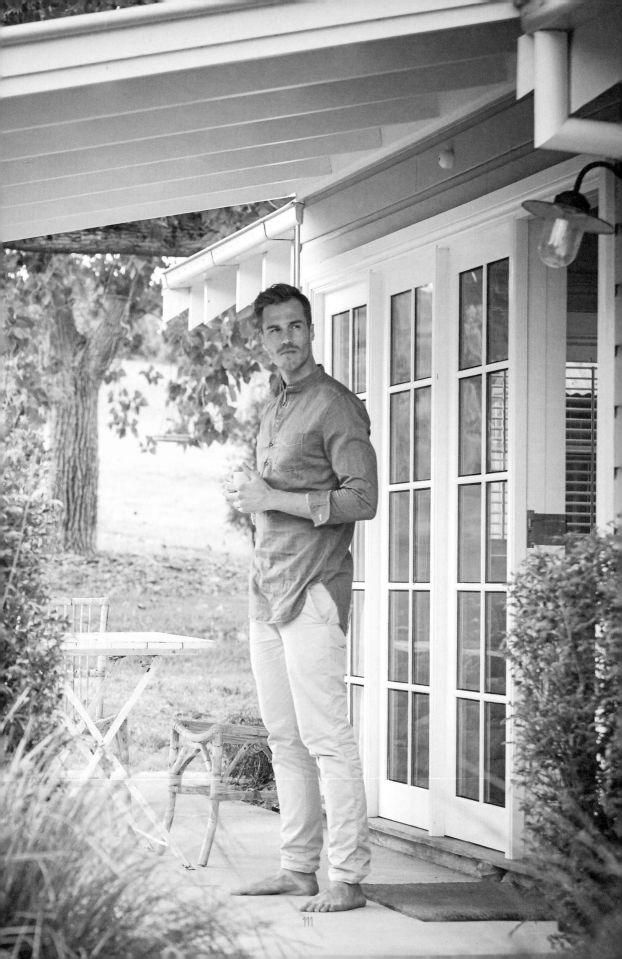

# DAILY RHYTHM

*A herbal approach to stress and sleep management*

**WE TALKED IN** the last chapter about the need for balance when it comes to stress management. A large part of that balance comes from what we do *after* we get home from work. A solid night's sleep leaves us refreshed to take on the next day like a champion, but a poor one leaves our minds tired and our bodies reluctant to work the way we wish they would.

Insomnia can be a complex and frustrating condition, and understanding why it happens to you is the first step in crafting a remedy that will lull you into a restful slumber. Is it anxious thoughts keeping you awake? Is your body stuck in 'fight-or-flight' mode and simply can't switch off? Or do you just not find yourself tired until after midnight, even though you know you've got a six o'clock wake-up call?

And that's just *sleep onset*. The next thing to work out is whether or not the sleep you're having is actually restorative. Are you waking up throughout the night? If so, you may be suffering from something called *poor sleep maintenance*.

Confused yet? Well my last question is this: are you dreaming? Dreams are a good indication that you are going through all the stages of deep sleep, but an interrupted, dreamless sleep might mean you're floating about in the shallows.

I remember when I was first taught about these different types and causes of insomnia, my head was spinning. I was in college, and my stress levels were at an all-time high. It was a senior student who was explaining this to me, as we stood in the student clinic, with bottles of tinctures stacked all around us. She was trying to convince me that I needed gentle *nervine* and *anxiolytic* herbs, rather than the high doses of *sedative* ones that I was adamant I needed

> Insomnia can be a complex and frustrating condition, and understanding why it happens to you is the first step in crafting a remedy that will lull you into a restful slumber.

> You'll likely find one or two 'hero remedies' out of this bunch that work better for you than the others. They're the herbs for you to stick to.

to chug. At first I resisted, and she almost had to pry the bottles out of my hands. I was certain that I just needed to have more of the strong mix I usually used.

Of course, she turned out to be right. A blissful blend of motherwort and passionflower became my new best friend. The gentle action of these herbs actually treated the cause of my poor sleep more effectively that the ones I normally used. It was a reminder of those old naturopathic philosophies: treat the cause, and treat the individual. After that, I made it my mission to learn about all things sleep-related, and the subtleties of herbal medicine in insomnia.

The following recipes cover all of the various elements that I described above. Some are outright sedative; others are more strongly nervine. One may help soothe the residues of the day's anxiety, while another might help you dive deeper into the depths of good sleep. You'll likely find one or two 'hero remedies' out of this bunch that work better for you than the others. They're the herbs for you to stick to.

## A NOTE ON MEDITATION

I would like to say I am a practised meditator but it's not the case. One thing that does help is my meditation candle. (See the recipe overleaf.)

The oil blend works just as effectively in an oil burner. If you're a master of aromatherapy you can mix up your own oils to create all kinds of therapeutic effects!

I light this candle while I practise deep-breathing exercises, as I'll admit to not being great at stilling my mind long enough to master meditation. Ensure you trim the wick each time before use, and Prue's hot tip is that it will burn more evenly if you give it a two-hour burn the first time you use it, but never to let it burn for more than four hours at a time.

# BEDTIME CHAI
## —for insomnia

Mum always said to have a glass of milk before bed, and she was right. Milk contains tryptophan, which our bodies convert into melatonin, our 'sleep hormone'. I've taken this classic mum's medicine, and ramped up its dream factor with a little *hypnotic* herb called valerian. Studies have shown that as little as 1 gram of this guy can induce relaxation and improve sleep onset. *Makes two serves.*

## YOU WILL NEED

**4 cardamom pods**

**1 cinnamon stick**

**3 teaspoons rooibos tea leaves**

**2–3 teaspoons finely chopped valerian root**

**1 vanilla bean pod, halved lengthwise**

**Large pinch of ground nutmeg**

**600 millilitres full-cream milk (or your favourite alternative *plus* 2 teaspoons coconut oil)**

**A little honey or stevia, to taste**

## HOW TO

**Step 1** Coarsely grind the cardamom pods and cinnamon stick in a coffee or spice grinder.

**Step 2** Place them in a heavy-based saucepan with the tea leaves, valerian root, whole vanilla bean pod and nutmeg.

**Step 3** Pour over the milk, plus the coconut oil if you're using a non-dairy option.

**Step 4** Bring to a simmer over a very low heat, stir well, then cover and continue to simmer for 8 minutes.

**Step 5** Remove from the heat and strain, discarding the solids.

**Step 6** Stir through your choice of sweetener if desired, then enjoy. Sweet dreams!

 Cardamom is called *ela* in Ayurvedic medicine, and has long been used to balance energy pathways. It's the perfect addition to this bedtime brew!

# MEDITATION CANDLE

## —to calm an anxious mind

This recipe actually comes from my sister Prue, who last year gave out handcrafted candles as gifts for guests at her wedding. I thought it was such a brilliant way to deliver aromatherapy that I asked her to teach me how to make them. You'll need to jump online to order a few special bits and bobs, but it's relatively inexpensive, and worth it if you think you'll be making a few of them. *Makes one candle that will burn for up to forty hours.*

## YOU WILL NEED

**For the 'zen' oil blend:**

**4 millilitres lavender essential oil**

**4 millilitres chamomile essential oil**

**For the candle:**

**'Wick Stick'em' double-sided sticker**

**15 cm waxed wick, with tab**

**Drinking straw**

**135 g soy wax**

**Wick holder (optional)**

**Kitchen or candy thermometer**

**7.9 x 6 cm apothecary jar**

## HOW TO

**Step 1** Combine your essential oils, and feel free to adjust the levels according to your preference.

**Step 2** Attach the double-sided sticker to the base of the wick tab. Run the wick through the drinking straw. Hold the clean jar upside down, and use the straw to press the wick tab firmly into place, centred at the base of the jar. Remove the straw.

**Step 3** Meanwhile, melt the wax in a bowl over a water bath on a low heat. Use the thermometer to keep an eye on the temperature, and once it's sitting between 65 and 70 degrees Celsius, remove from the heat.

**Step 4** Add your essential oil, keeping an eye on the temperature of the mix. You want it sitting between 60 and 65 degrees when you pour it into the jar. Stir well to make sure your fragrance is evenly dispersed.

**Step 5** Prepare the jar by placing it upright on a sheet of newspaper or absorbent paper. Use the aptly named wick holder by placing it over the mouth of the jar, with the wick running through the hole and securing it in place. This keeps the wick straight and taut while we fill the candle. In a pinch, a pair of chopsticks and some sticky tape will do the same job.

**Step 6** Slowly pour the wax and oil mix into the jar, being careful to fill the glass evenly to avoid bubbles. Leave the candle where it is to set over twenty-four hours, then trim the wick down to 1 centimetre before use.

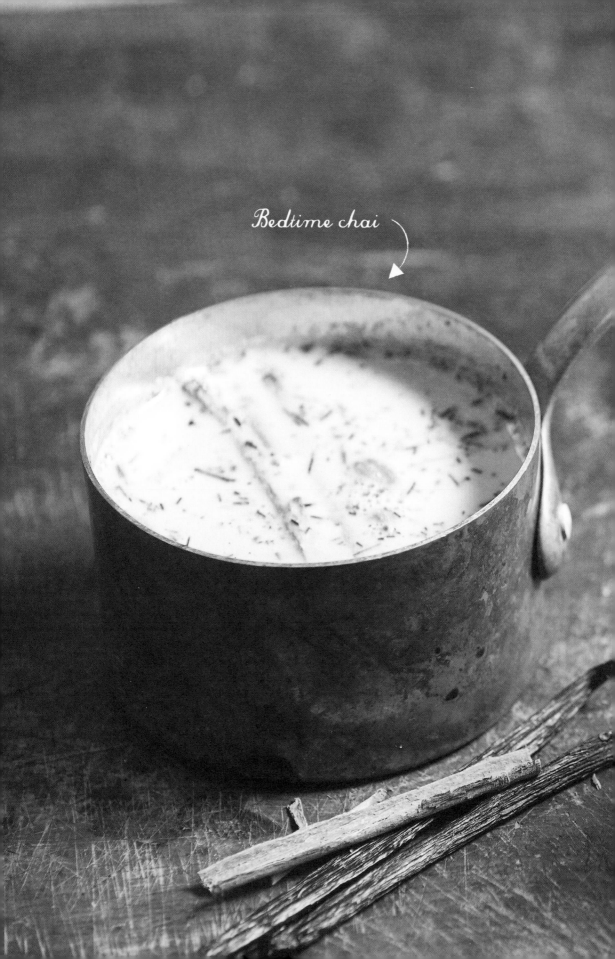

Bedtime chai

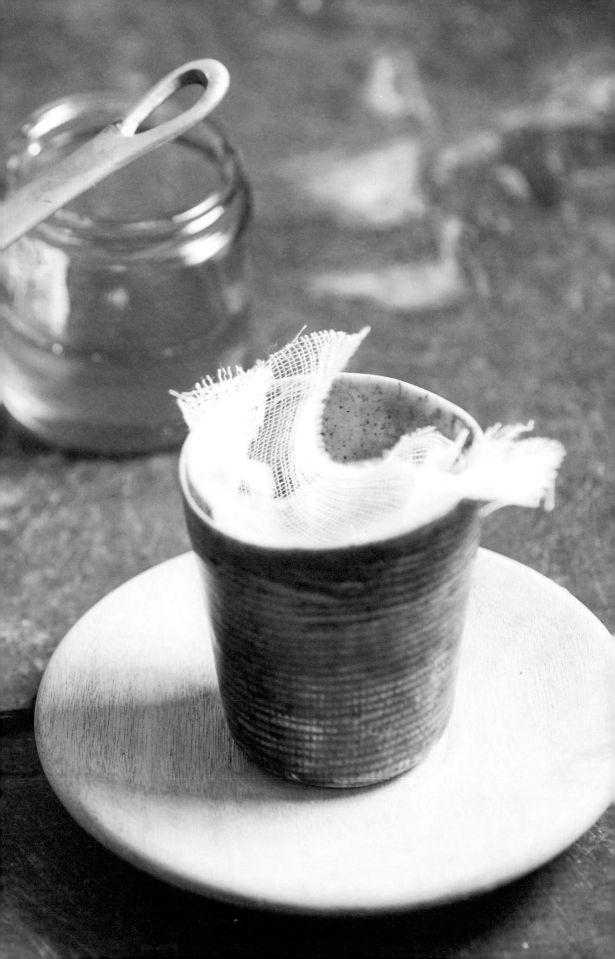

# 'CHILL PILL' BATH BOMB

## —to relax and unwind

Go home, turn your phone off and soak your day away in a hot bath. Lavender contains linalool, a substance that's been shown in studies to reduce the physical signs of stress. It's my favourite anti-anxiety herb, and you can enjoy the benefits just by smelling it!

The citric acid and the bicarbonate of soda create an acid-base reaction that you may remember from school, and that's what gives these bath bombs their fizz. *Makes one.*

## YOU WILL NEED

**9 teaspoons bicarbonate of soda**

**3 teaspoons citric acid**

**1 teaspoon dried lavender**

**10–20 drops lavender essential oil**

**1 teaspoon sweet almond oil**

## HOW TO

**Step 1** Ensure your small mixing bowl and spoon are dry, otherwise you'll set off the bubbling early.

**Step 2** Combine the dry ingredients and mix thoroughly.

**Step 3** Add the oils and knead the mixture together using the back of a spoon. It will form a very dry, crumbly paste.

**Step 4** Spoon the mixture into a muffin cup and leave it somewhere warm to dry for at least an hour. Then you can gently remove it from the mould.

**Step 5** Pop one into the bath and let your stresses melt away!

 **HERB NERD HACK** If you are going to make a few of these at once and store them, be sure to keep them wrapped in aluminium foil to keep them from drying out.

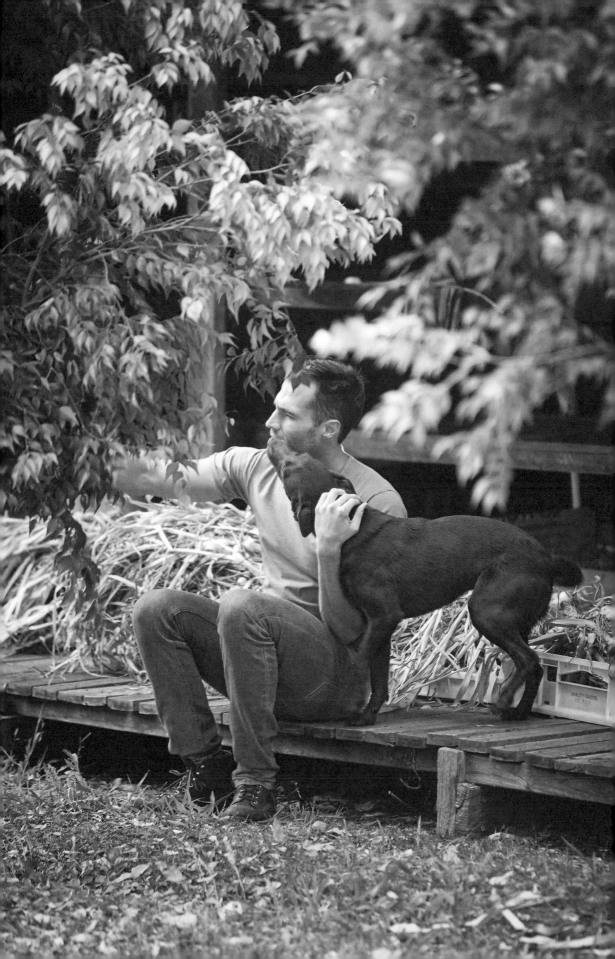

# Herbal Teas

Herbal teas are one of my favourite ways to administer medicines that combat stress. Why? Because the very action of stopping what you're doing and brewing a tea is in itself therapeutic; it's a ritual for giving yourself permission to relax and unwind. The process of brewing a tea is like saying to yourself 'I deserve down time,' and honouring your need for rest and recovery.

So that's how I want you to think of these tea blends. Create a big batch of your favourite, and keep it on hand for whenever you need to press pause on your frantic day. All of these can be made in bulk, and stored in airtight jars until needed.

# MUM'S BEST MATE
## —for mothers and carers

There is something about the combination of passionflower and motherwort that is a little bit magical. I was first introduced to it during the clinical portion of my degree, and thought it was an odd recommendation—after all, it's motherwort's traditional use as a tonic for wearied mothers that earned it its name, and I'm obviously not a mother!

I was assured that it is a worthy addition to the herbal treatment of anyone whose energy is depleted from caring for others. Nurses, teachers and other carers would all benefit from a little motherwort at the end of the day, during a tea break or—in the case of kindergarten teachers—maybe even during nap time.

## YOU WILL NEED

**1 cup dried motherwort**
**1 cup dried passionflower**
**1 handful dried rose petals**

## HOW TO

Combine the herbs and petals well, and use one or two teaspoons in a cup of boiled water. Infuse for 5–6 minutes, then strain and enjoy.

# 6 PM BLEND
## —wave goodbye to the work day

It seems like work is encroaching further and further into our private lives. We stay late, take our work home with us and even allow it to creep into the bedroom through our phones and ever-bleeping emails. There's no doubt that it's a contributing factor in disrupted circadian rhythm and that feeling of never being able to switch off. So it's high time that we took a stand and reclaimed our evenings as our own. Enjoy a mug of this blend in place of a wine at the end of the day, then make a promise to yourself to put work aside until the next morning. You'll thank me.

## YOU WILL NEED

1 ½ **cups dried lemon balm**

½ **cup dried chamomile**

**1 tablespoon dried lavender**

## HOW TO

Combine all of the ingredients and mix well. You can use anywhere up to a tablespoon of this mix per mug as an infusion.

# NOURISH AND NURTURE
## —for feelings of exhaustion

If you feel you've pushed your body to the point of no return, are tired even after a solid night's sleep and can't muster the energy to get up and go, this might just be the blend for you. You'll need to make it a part of your daily routine to really see the benefits, but avoid this one if you have high blood pressure.

## YOU WILL NEED

**2 cups dried licorice root**

**1 tablespoon dried lavender**

## HOW TO

Combine the two herbs, and mix well. You'll need to make a decoction of this one (see page 63) using around two teaspoons of the mix in each cup.

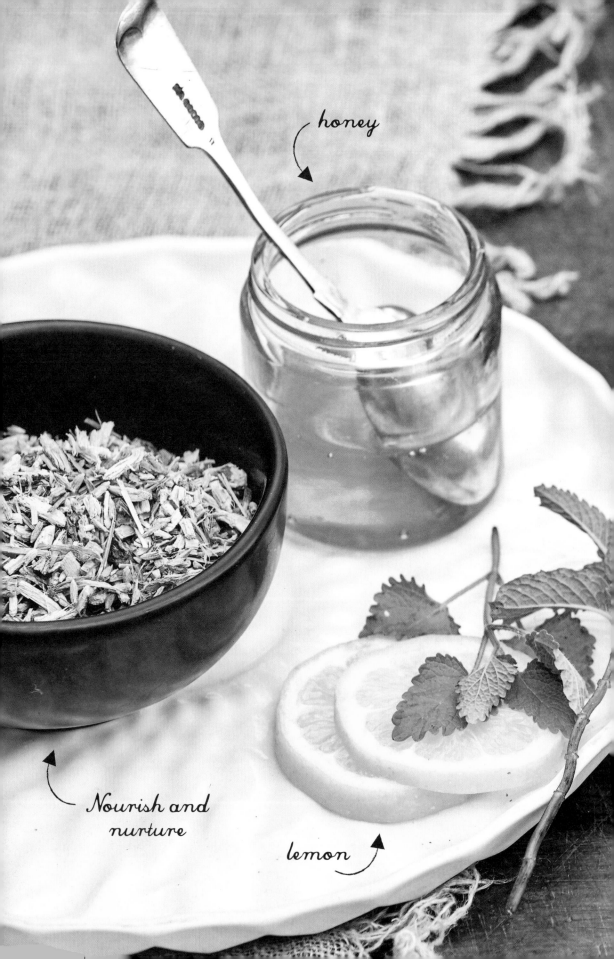

honey

Nourish and
nurture

lemon

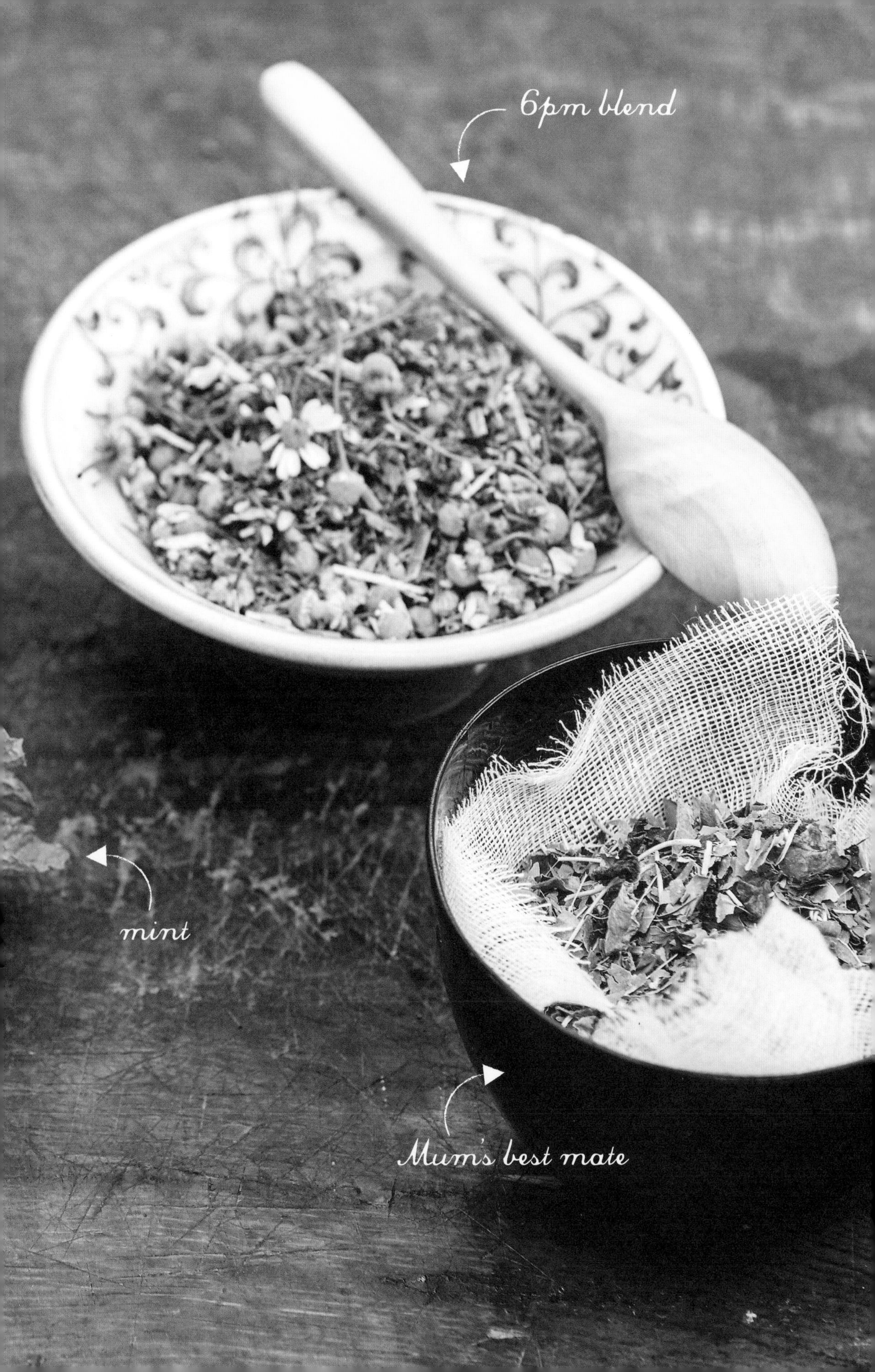

6pm blend

mint

Mum's best mate

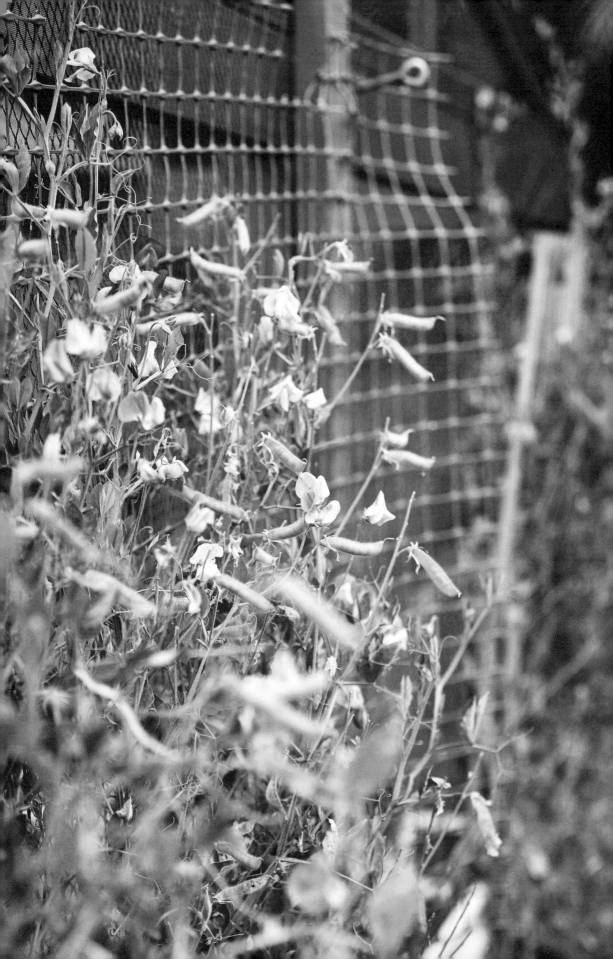

# Lemon Balm Iced Tea

## —for stress

It's all too easy to reach for the bottle of pinot at the end of a hard day at work, and every now and again that won't hurt you. But regular drinking has been linked to so many health conditions that you'd be better off keeping it for special occasions, and instead turning to the herb patch when stress strikes. Lemon balm is one of my favourite *nervine* herbs, meaning that it balances an overactive nervous system, and it is so simple to grow that I'd almost go as far as to say that everyone should have it in their garden.

This sparkling iced tea is the perfect way to enjoy it, and is particularly good on a warm day. *The recipe just makes one drink, but feel free to make a whole pitcher and enjoy it with friends.*

## YOU WILL NEED

**For the infusion:**

**Handful fresh lemon balm (10–15 leaves)**

**Handful fresh mint (10–15 leaves)**

**1 teaspoon honey, or a pinch of stevia**

**1 slice of lemon**

**Boiling water, to cover**

**To serve:**

**Glassful of ice**

**Extra lemon slices and a sprig of mint, to garnish**

**Soda water, to top up**

## HOW TO

**Step 1** Crush the lemon balm and mint leaves in a mortar and pestle, then transfer to a shallow bowl or ramekin.

**Step 2** Add the honey (or stevia) plus the lemon slice, and pour over just enough boiling water to cover the mix. We want to make this infusion very concentrated, so don't overdo the water.

**Step 3** Cover, and leave to infuse for 5–8 minutes. Meanwhile, fill your serving glass with ice, and arrange the mint sprig and lemon slices.

**Step 4** Strain the infusion and pour over the ice.

**Step 5** Top up the glass with cold soda water, and you're ready to kick back and enjoy!

 **HERB NERD HACK** A couple of fresh lavender heads make a wonderful addition to this mix if you like the flavour, or if you don't have any lemon balm you can substitute chamomile for a more floral taste.

# Sleep Potion
## —for insomnia

Around 90 per cent of the people who come through my clinic doors will tell me that, at some point, they've had trouble sleeping. It's one of the most common complaints I see, and one that prompts the most gratitude when it's resolved. A well-crafted herbal tincture for sleep contains not just *sedative* herbs, but *anxiolytic* ones too. Anxiolytic, you can probably decipher, indicates that a herb is used to reduce feelings of anxiety. I find this to be an important addition because for many people who already feel tired, it's the recurring worries from their busy day that plague their mind and prevent proper sleep patterns.

This blend takes into account both of those actions, so that it does more than just make you feel sleepy; it also lifts the stress of the day from your shoulders, removing the road blocks to a peaceful night's sleep.

## YOU WILL NEED

**25 g dried hops**
**50 g dried passionflower**
**75 g dried ashwaganda**
**500 millilitres (2 cups) vodka**

## HOW TO

**Step 1** Grind the three herbs in a coffee or spice grinder, and transfer to a large sterile jar.

**Step 2** Add the vodka, replace the lid and shake well.

**Step 3** Place the jar in a cool, dark place for two weeks. Each day, go and shake the jar gently to keep the herbs from settling.

**Step 4** After two weeks, strain the mixture through cheesecloth and discard the solids. You may need to wear gloves and squeeze nice and hard to get the most extract out of your mix. Pour the tincture into a clean jar.

**Step 5** Take six teaspoons (that's 30 millilitres in total) in a little water, about an hour before bed.

 **HERB NERD HACK** A nice way to dose this one is by pouring yourself a cup of boiled water and adding the tincture. Let some of the alcohol evaporate off before stirring through a little honey or stevia.

Note: If you prefer to make an alcohol-free version of this remedy, please use the glycetract method (see page 58).

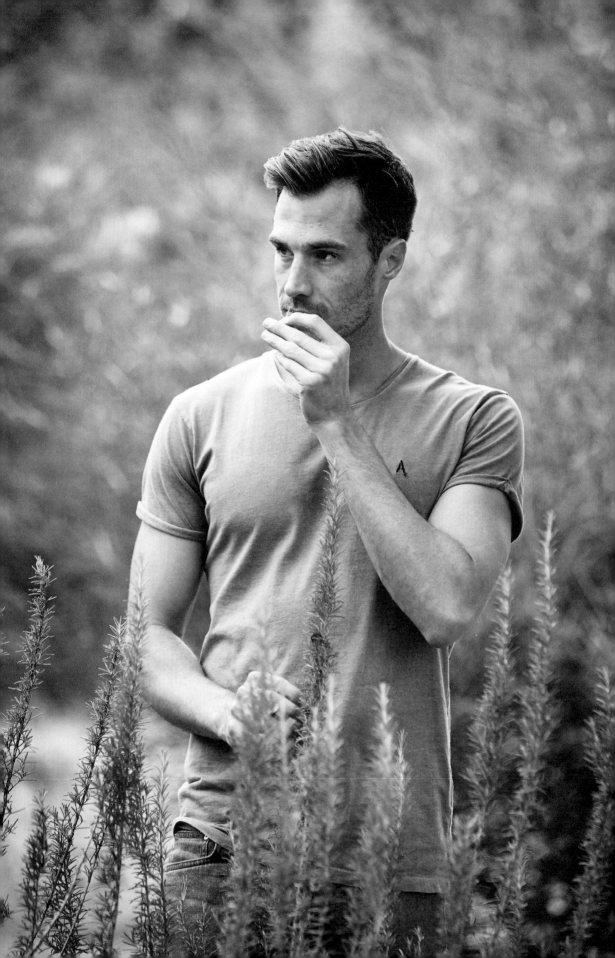

THE USE OF
HONEY AS A
MEDICINE FOR
TISSUE REPAIR
EXTENDS AS
FAR BACK AS
ANCIENT EGYPT,
AND POSSIBLY
FURTHER.

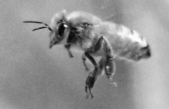

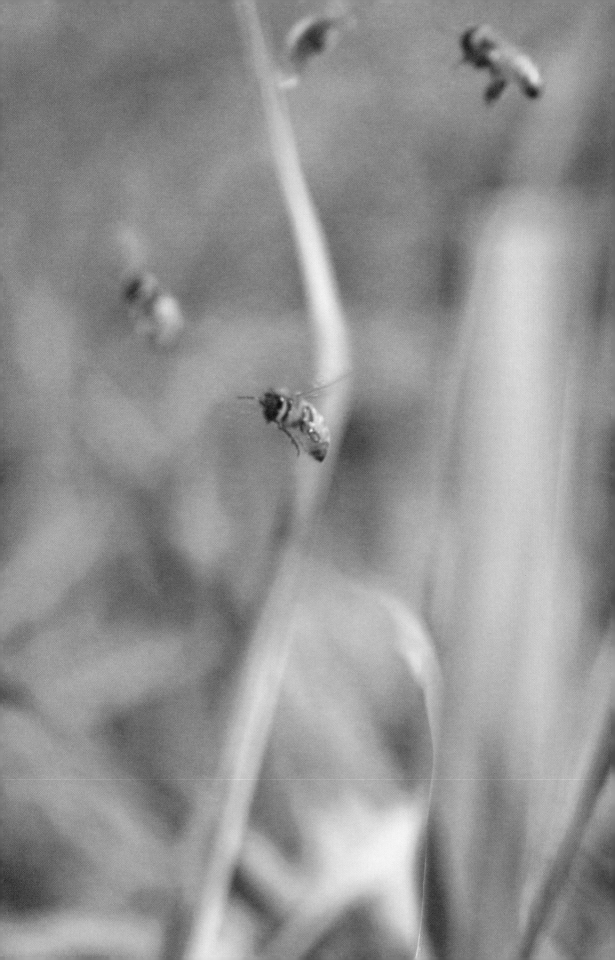

# GUT INSTINCT

*Your guide to bloating, indigestion and other tummy troubles*

**THERE'S THIS OLD** naturopathic concept called the gut–brain axis. For a long time it was shrugged off and barely understood, but as modern science catches up with ancient wisdom, we are finding more and more links between gut health and mental wellbeing. Not just that, but it looks like gut health affects all of the other systems in the body too!

After all, we may be made up of a bunch of systems—nervous, circulatory, respiratory, among others—but ultimately they still form one organism: the human one. And that organism plays host to billions of microscopic inhabitants that form one very special ecosystem, with each part of it affecting another. It makes sense then, that when our digestive system isn't happy, other parts of our health will suffer too.

For example, did you know that between 70 and 90 per cent of our serotonin (the 'antidepressant hormone') is located in the digestive system, and not the brain as you might imagine? Or that an imbalance of gut bacteria has been linked to chronic autoimmune conditions? Or perhaps, on a more day-to-day scale, you've noticed how you need to run to the bathroom more often when you're nervous? All of these things are examples of just how intricately our gut is linked to every other part of our body, and why we should be paying attention when it cries for help with bloating, pain or indigestion.

Long-term wear and tear on the digestive system—whether it be from food intolerances, infection or overuse of alcohol and medications—leads to an inflamed gut lining. Your hyper-reactive gut then becomes sensitive to foods that normally wouldn't pose any problem for you, and the inflammation worsens. The whole scenario snowballs, and usually results in

> We are finding more and more links between gut health and mental wellbeing.

an increasingly restrictive diet to manage your digestive discomfort. But removing the offending foods is only one part of the treatment, and actively repairing your damaged digestive system should form a core part of correcting the problem.

You may even find, with time, that you can reintroduce some of the foods you cut out, and without a nasty backlash from your gut!

For example, take a common herbal hero of the gut, slippery elm. While it's often used to treat heartburn, it doesn't actually neutralise stomach acid like your pharmacy brands of antacid do. Rather, it coats the irritated lining of the stomach and oesophagus, symptomatically treating the pain without reducing your acid levels or digestive capacity.

It wouldn't be a gut health chapter without a mention of fermented foods, so check out the hibiscus and raspberry kefir recipe on page 137. More and more research shows that the human body is in

Long-term wear and tear on the digestive system leads to an inflamed gut lining.

fact an entire ecosystem, and that a happy gut microbiota (that's the population of friendly bacteria that live inside your tummy) regulates everything from digestion to mental health and even immunity. The actual balancing act in the gut is a very complex one, but daily consumption of probiotic foods like kefir certainly helps to promote a healthy 'human ecosystem'.

# ANTI-INFLAMMITEA
## —for IBS, bloating and joint pain

This tea is more like a chai: milky and richly spiced. It is so delicious that it's easy to forget that you are taking your medicine. But with a formidable line-up of anti-inflammatory ingredients, this bright yellow indulgence is a go-to rescue remedy for any kind of long-term tummy troubles. Bloating, cramps and irritable bowel syndrome (IBS) might all benefit from a little anti-inflammitea.

Curcumin, a heavily researched compound found in turmeric, is the star ingredient here, and the addition of black pepper is known to help it cross into the bloodstream so that it can work its magic in other parts of the body. I even have one friend who swears by this for her arthritis! *Makes one.*

## YOU WILL NEED

**6–8 cm piece of fresh turmeric**

**3–4 cm piece of fresh ginger**

**1 cinnamon stick**

**1 teaspoon cardamom pods**

**1 pinch of black pepper**

**1 teaspoon black tea (or contents of one tea bag)**

**250 millilitres (1 cup) full-cream milk (or your favourite dairy substitute)**

**250 millilitres (1 cup) filtered water**

**Manuka honey, to taste**

## HOW TO

**Step 1** Peel and then finely grate the ginger and turmeric.

**Step 2** Grind your dried spices in a coffee or spice grinder.

**Step 3** Place all of the ingredients except the honey into a large saucepan and bring to a boil, then reduce the heat to very low.

**Step 4** Simmer for 10 minutes, being careful not to let it boil over.

**Step 5** Remove from the heat and strain the mixture, discarding the solids.

**Step 6** Sweeten with manuka honey and enjoy! Can be consumed daily for optimal effect.

 **HERB NERD HACK** Manuka is believed to coat the linings of irritated tummy tissues and support their healing.

# A Digestive Decoction

## —for indigestion

So you overindulged at dinnertime and are left feeling sore and bloated. If you've got a well-stocked pantry and a little pot of peppermint, you've got everything you need to make a quick-fix remedy on the spot. A quick trip to the garden and a look through the spice rack will see you with three very effective ingredients that can be whipped up to make a therapeutic cuppa. *This recipe makes one drink, but feel free to increase the amounts to make a pot of tea to share—if all your guests overdid it too!*

## YOU WILL NEED

**½ teaspoon dried fennel seeds**

**1 teaspoon dried licorice root**

**500 millilitres (2 cups) water**

**Handful of fresh peppermint (15–20 leaves)**

## HOW TO

**Step 1** Give your fennel seeds a quick grind in the mortar and pestle to release the oils. Pour them into a heavy-based saucepan along with the licorice root.

**Step 2** Add the water and bring to a boil over a high heat.

**Step 3** Cover with a lid, and leave on high heat to decoct for 5 minutes.

**Step 4** Meanwhile, crush the peppermint leaves lightly in the mortar and pestle.

**Step 5** Turn off the heat, throw the peppermint into the pot, stir through and replace the lid.

**Step 6** Leave for another 5 minutes, then strain into a cup for immediate enjoyment!

Note: As delicious as licorice is, it can slightly raise blood pressure in susceptible individuals, so give this a miss if you know yours is a little high already.

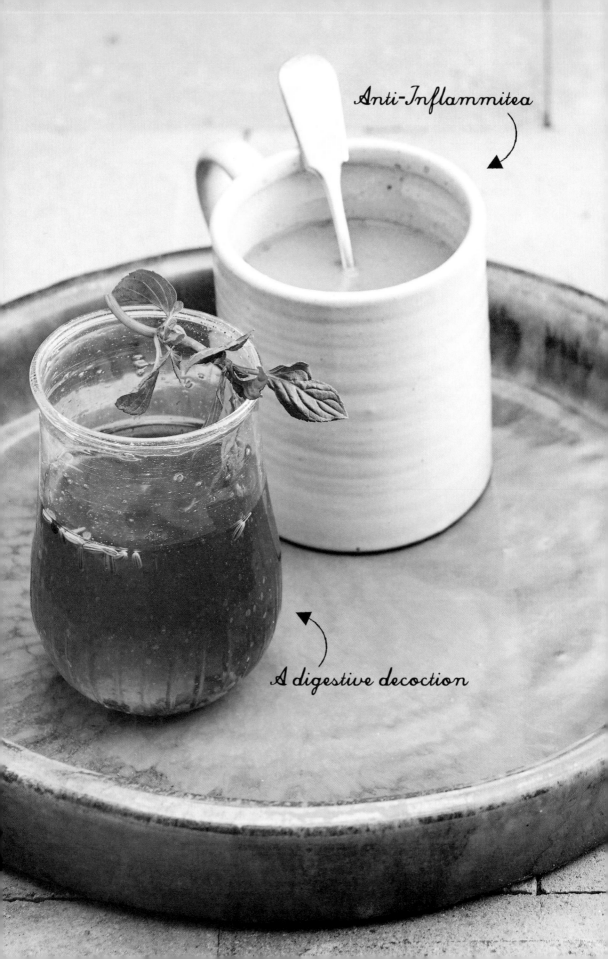

Anti-Inflammitea

A digestive decoction

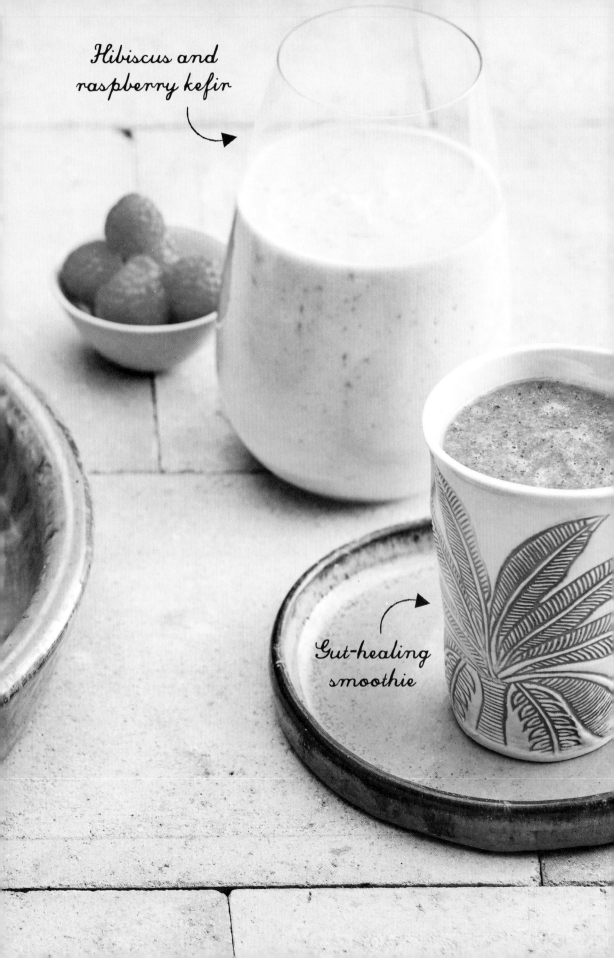

Hibiscus and
raspberry kefir

Gut-healing
smoothie

# GUT-HEALING SMOOTHIE
## —for IBS and leaky gut

Aloe vera and slippery elm have long been used to coat and soothe a suffering digestive system, while peppermint is known as a *carminative* herb, easing the passage of food. Kiwifruit contains an enzyme called actinidain, which itself assists with protein digestion. Besides, kiwi and mint is a delicious combo! *Makes one smoothie.*

## YOU WILL NEED

**1 medium aloe vera leaf**

**½ teaspoon slippery elm bark powder**

**10–12 fresh peppermint leaves**

**2 ripe kiwifruit, peeled and roughly chopped**

**Small handful baby spinach leaves**

**10 cm length of cucumber, peeled and roughly chopped**

**250 millilitres (1 cup) coconut water**

## HOW TO

**Step 1** Carefully slice off the top layer of skin from the aloe leaf. Using a spoon, gently scoop out the gel, being careful not to get any of the green fibres.

**Step 2** Place gel in a blender with the remaining ingredients and blend until smooth.

**Step 3** Serve in a tall glass, and enjoy!

 **HERB NERD HACK** Pineapple and papaya contain similar enzymes to kiwifruit, so feel free to alternate between your favourite of the three fruits, depending on taste and seasonal availability.

# HIBISCUS AND RASPBERRY KEFIR

## —for healthy gut bacteria

Kefir is a Turkish drinkable yoghurt and is probably the easiest introduction to fermented foods. You can pick up the starter culture—called 'grains' even though they're not grains at all—cheaply at most health food stores. Hibiscus gives it a deep pink colour, and delivers a dose of herbal goodness for tissue repair. My only advice is not to cook with it, as the heat will kill off some of the bacteria and render it less potent.

The raspberries will shorten the shelf life of this product, so you'll want to polish it off within four or five days. *Makes approximately four half-cup serves.*

## YOU WILL NEED

**500 millilitres (2 cups) coconut milk (or full-cream milk if you can tolerate dairy)**

**1 teaspoon kefir 'grains'**

**2 tablespoons dried hibiscus (rosella) petals**

**¼ cup fresh raspberries**

## HOW TO

**Step 1**  In a sterile glass jar, combine the milk and kefir grains.

**Step 2**  Stir well, then cover with cheesecloth, kept in place with an elastic band.

**Step 3**  Store at room temperature (around 20 degrees Celsius) for 24–48 hours.

**Step 4**  Stir through the hibiscus, replace the cheesecloth cover, and leave in the fridge overnight to infuse.

**Step 5**  Strain the mixture, and discard the solids.

**Step 6**  Transfer the kefir to a blender, add raspberries and blitz until smooth.

**Step 7**  Pour into a sterile glass jar, seal with the lid and keep in the fridge. Shake well before each use, as it may separate in the bottle.

 **HERB NERD HACK**  You can get more bang for your buck by removing half a cup of the kefir before adding the hibiscus, and using it as a starter culture for a new batch!

# GINGER PASTILLES
## —for nausea

Nausea? Ginger. Hangover? Ginger. Motion sickness? Ginger. This cousin to turmeric is the best *anti-emetic,* or 'tummy settler', going around. But let's face it: we don't always have the time to stop and put on a pot of tea. Keep a little container of these in the fridge if you suspect you may need them, and suck on a pastille as required. *Makes twelve.*

## YOU WILL NEED

**For the tincture:**

**30 g dried ginger**

**120 millilitres vodka**

**For the pastilles:**

**60 millilitres ginger tincture (from recipe above)**

**24 g powdered gelatine (or agar-agar)**

**24 millilitres vegetable glycerine**

**24 millilitres water**

**coconut oil, to coat moulds**

## HOW TO

**Step 1**  Grind the ginger in a coffee or spice grinder until you have a fine powder. Pour into a sterile jar; cover with the vodka.

**Step 2**  Leave for two weeks, then strain through cheesecloth. You may find you have significantly more tincture than the 60 millilitres that is required for the pastilles, but it's better to have too much than too little. If you made more than you need, you can keep the extra for something else.

**Step 3**  Combine everything but the tincture in a bowl and heat over a water bath until melted. Remove from the heat.

**Step 4**  Measure out 60 millilitres of your ginger tincture and stir it through the melted ingredients.

**Step 5**  Shallow pour into an ice cube tray (you may need to coat with a little coconut oil first) and leave pastilles to set in the fridge.

**Step 6**  Once set, carefully cut them into 1 cm x 2 cm pieces, and wrap in greaseproof paper. Store in the fridge, and use within a week.

 **If you find the ginger knocks your socks off and is too strong, halve the ginger used in the tincture recipe to get a softer 1:8 remedy. More details on making tinctures can be found on page 54.**

Note: Although ginger is a common remedy for morning sickness, I actually don't recommend you have these during pregnancy. Stick to a weak ginger tea instead.

# NATURE'S ANTACID PILLS
## —for heartburn

The process of making these guys is long and slow, but the end result is a jar of very convenient, homemade capsules that you can take anywhere with you. If you like the idea, but aren't so keen on the amount of time it takes to do this manually, you can buy small capsule machines that make this job a little easier. The empty capsules themselves are readily available online, or in good health food stores. *Makes twenty-four capsules.*

## YOU WILL NEED

**20 g slippery elm powder**

**24 VegeCap empty capsules (size one)**

## HOW TO

**Step 1** Place your powdered slippery elm into a bowl.

**Step 2** Scoop up as much as you can into the longer end of the empty capsule.

**Step 3** Using a clean chopstick, press the herb down.

**Step 4** Add more powder, and tamp down again. Continue to do this until it's filled.

**Step 5** Slide the other end of the capsule into place.

**Step 6** Repeat the process for all of the capsules, then store in a clean, dry, amber glass jar.

**Step 7** Take two capsules at a time, anywhere up to three times daily for relief.

 **You can use this same method to make dried turmeric capsules, and use them as a natural anti-inflammatory.**

Note: Take these ones a few hours after any other medication you have, as they may slow absorption.

Nature's antacid
pills

Peppermint belly jellies

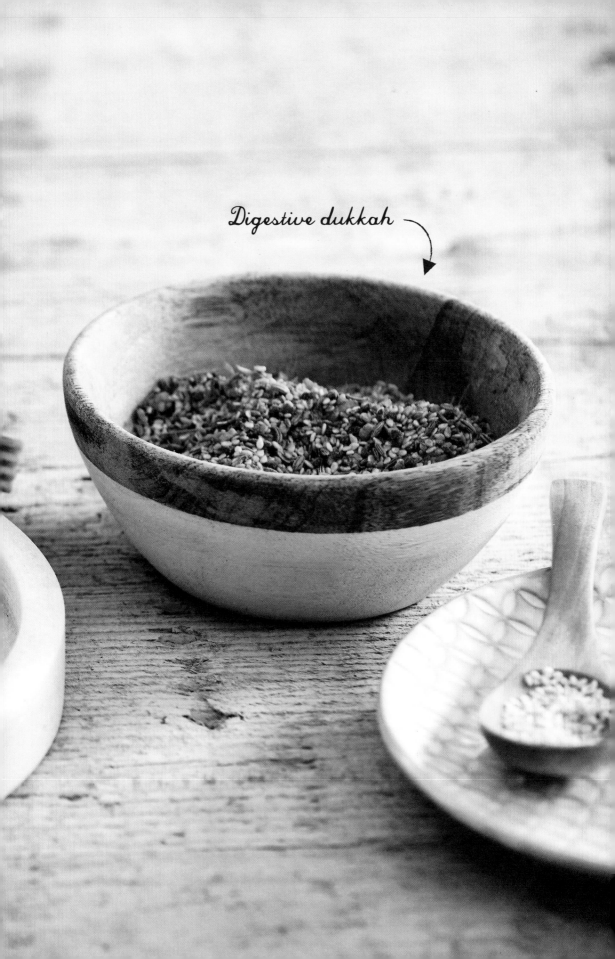

Digestive dukkah

# DIGESTIVE DUKKAH
## —for bloating

Fennel seeds contain oils that relax the muscle lining our digestive tract. The seeds can ease digestion and help relieve painful bloating. I find that this dukkah is an easy remedy for those prone to bloating because it is delicious sprinkled on almost anything. The addition of turmeric adds an anti-inflammatory twist to this spice mix, making it a worthy addition to the diets of those who have been suffering tummy troubles for far too long. *Makes approximately two-thirds of a cup.*

## YOU WILL NEED

¼ cup raw almonds

6 teaspoons dried cumin seeds

6 teaspoons dried coriander seeds

3 teaspoons dried fennel seeds

3 teaspoons dried turmeric

4 teaspoons white sesame seeds

3 teaspoons black sesame seeds

sea salt and freshly ground black pepper, to taste

## HOW TO

**Step 1** Start by spreading out the almonds in a baking tray, then roast for 8–10 minutes in a medium oven (180 degrees Celsius). Leave to cool.

**Step 2** Meanwhile, place the cumin and coriander seeds in a dry frying pan and heat over a high heat until fragrant. Shake the pan every so often to keep them moving and cooking on all sides.

**Step 3** Pour the cumin, coriander and fennel seeds into a coffee or spice grinder. Careful not to overdo it; you want them to still resemble fragments of the original spices, and not grind them all the way to a powder.

**Step 4** Chop the almonds into small pieces, then place them in a bowl with the ground spices.

**Step 5** Stir through the turmeric and sesame seeds.

**Step 6** Taste, then season with salt and pepper.

## HOW DO I USE IT?

Soft-boil two eggs, then carefully peel away the shells and coat the eggs in olive oil. Roll the eggs in the dukkah, then serve with blanched asparagus for a quick, healthy breakfast or lunch!

# Belly Jellies
## —to make your tummy smile

These delicious jellies can be moulded into fun shapes like gummy bears and snakes. Silicone moulds work best and are available online or at kitchen stores, but you can also just line a shallow baking tray, pour the mix into one large mould, then cut it into squares once set.

If you're vegetarian or vegan, you can use an equal amount of agar-agar in place of gelatine, but you will need to bring your liquid up to a boil again once you've added the powder (or it won't combine properly).

Store your jellies in an airtight container in the fridge and use them up within a week. *Makes approximately 18–20 jellies.*

## Hibiscus and Orange Blossom Jellies

Hibiscus has a reputation for aiding tissue repair. So if the peppermint flavour belly jellies are for a quick fix, these gummies are more about long-term repair—yes, that means I'm giving you permission to make these a daily thing!

### YOU WILL NEED

**300 millitres water**

**6 teaspoons dried hibiscus (rosella) petals**

**12–16 drops stevia extract**

**6 teaspoons orange blossom water**

**9 teaspoons (45 millilitres) gelatine (or agar-agar)**

### HOW TO

**Step 1** Bring the water to a boil in a saucepan over a medium heat.

**Step 2** Turn off the heat, stir through the hibiscus petals and cover.

**Step 3** After 5 minutes, strain your mix and discard the solids.

**Step 4** Measure out 200 millilitres of the hibiscus infusion, and add the stevia and orange blossom water. Give it a quick stir.

**Step 5** Whisk the gelatine through with a fork, then pour into your mould or moulds.

**Step 6** Place in the fridge and leave for 1 to 2 hours or until completely set.

# Peppermint Belly Jellies

As you've probably already realised by now, I'm a big fan of peppermint for digestion. It's one of the best carminatives—that means it relaxes the gut lining and eases digestion—which we have, so it is perfect to keep in the herbal first aid kit. Pull these jellies out as a cute after-dinner treat for your guests.

Because the active constituent is an oil it is more soluble in fat, so you'll see more benefit from using coconut milk or a full-cream milk in this recipe rather than water. You do have the option of straining the herb out of the mix before letting it set, but in the name of getting the most benefit out of your herb, I recommend leaving it in.

## YOU WILL NEED

**300 millilitres coconut milk**

**1 cup fresh peppermint leaves**.

**12–16 drops stevia extract**

**9 teaspoons (45 millilitres) gelatine (or agar-agar)**

## HOW TO

**Step 1** Put the coconut milk and peppermint leaves into a blender and blend until smooth.

**Step 2** Pour into a heavy-based saucepan and bring to a boil over a medium heat. Turn the heat off, and leave to infuse with the lid on for 5 minutes.

**Step 3** Stir through the stevia extract.

**Step 4** Whisk the gelatine or agar-agar through with a fork, then pour into your mould or moulds.

**Step 5** Place in the fridge for 1 to 2 hours or until completely set. Enjoy!

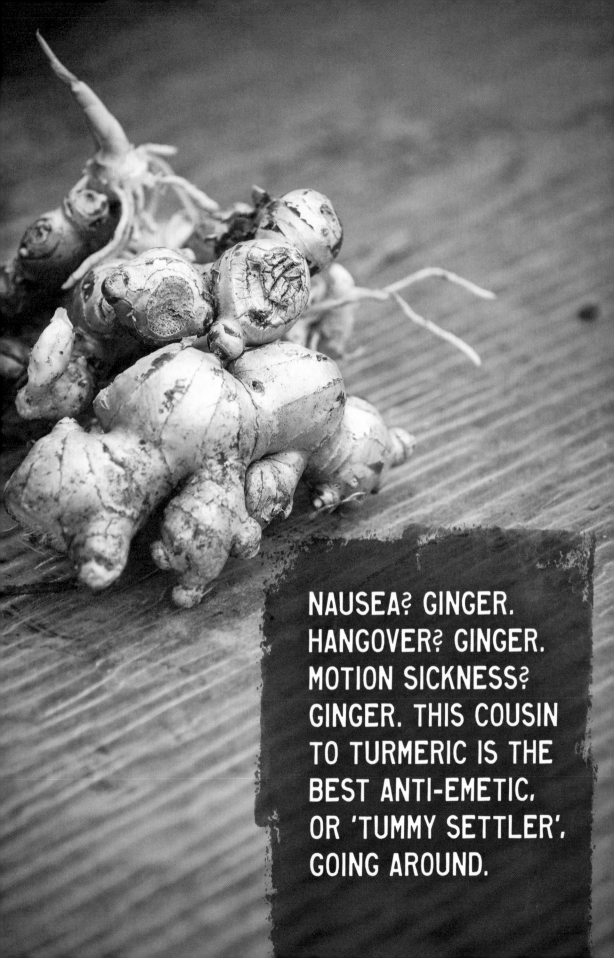

NAUSEA? GINGER.
HANGOVER? GINGER.
MOTION SICKNESS?
GINGER. THIS COUSIN
TO TURMERIC IS THE
BEST ANTI-EMETIC,
OR 'TUMMY SETTLER',
GOING AROUND.

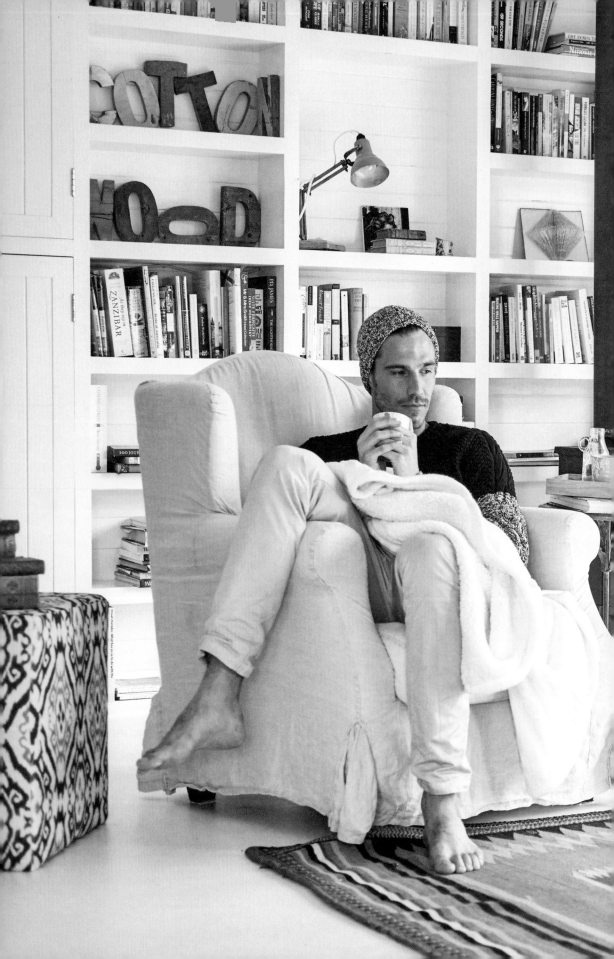

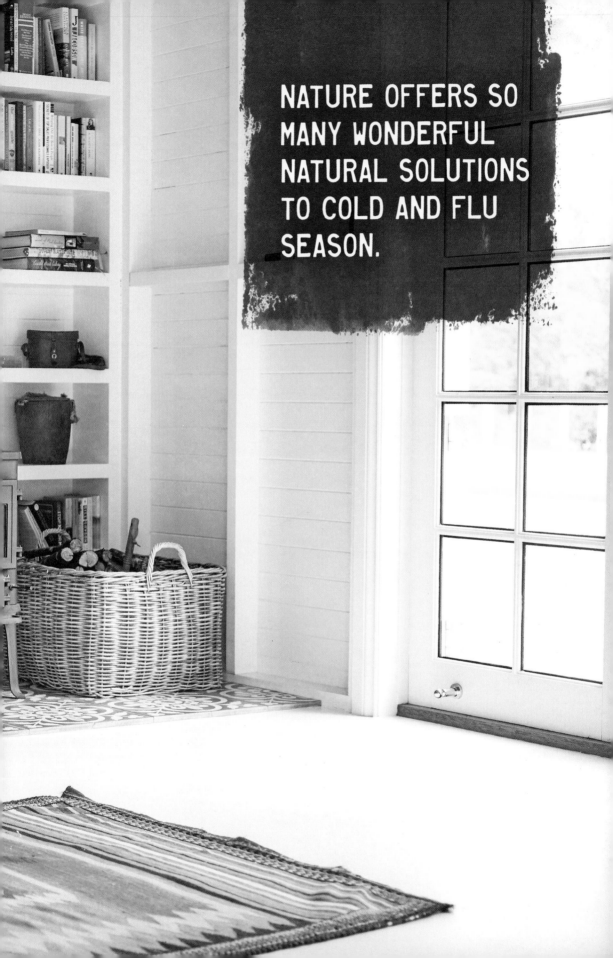

NATURE OFFERS SO MANY WONDERFUL NATURAL SOLUTIONS TO COLD AND FLU SEASON.

# FLU FIGHTERS

*Immune system tonics for colds, flus and allergies*

**TURNING SCEPTICS AROUND** is one of my favourite pastimes. All of my friends have been supportive (and often very patient) with my eccentricities and weird herbal habits, but not all of them have believed that herbal medicine could be nearly as effective as it is. I derive great pleasure, then, when my friends get sick. Don't take that the wrong way, I don't like to see them ill! Rather, I love the opportunity to swoop in with a customised tincture and get them back to health.

I remember when two friends of mine who also happened to be housemates were both home from work, coughing and sneezing on the couch. I delivered two bottles of my most potent brew, and instructed them how to take it. One followed my instructions; the other did not. Guess who got better first?

Another time, I had a friend come to me who had battled lifelong allergies. He was open to trying the natural approach, but didn't hold much hope for its success.

'Don't worry if it doesn't work', he said, 'nothing has ever really worked for me'.

Those words sent me into herb nerd overdrive. I wasn't going to let any allergy get the better of me, and made it my mission to concoct a remedy that would decrease his allergic response, dry up his sinuses and blast out anything that was blocking them. My friend became so in love with the mix that, even when he moved overseas, he continued to ask me to send it to him. It gave him, in his own words, 'almost complete resolution. I can breathe'!

Immune system tonics are wonderful remedies to show off your newfound herbal skills to friends and family, partly because the effect is noticeable almost immediately. Make up big batches of your favourites at the start of winter—or at the start of hay fever season in spring—and get ready to share them. Prepare yourself to be very popular!

> Immune system tonics are wonderful remedies to show off your newfound herbal skills to friends and family

# SORE THROAT SPRAY
## —for dry or productive sore throats

Sore throat remedies require a few different herbal actions. *Demulcent* (which basically means 'tissue soothing') herbs make up a large part of it, soothing the area; expectorants help your body expel annoying build-up; circulatory stimulating ingredients help increase blood flow to the area to support natural healing; and *antimicrobial* herbs fight off the bugs. I've included herbs that cover all of these actions to make a handy spray you can carry around with you, for when you need it most.

## YOU WILL NEED

**50 millilitres water**

**3 teaspoons food-grade vegetable glycerine**

**2 teaspoons each of 1:4 strength licorice, marshmallow, ginger, thyme and calendula tinctures**

Note: You'll need to already have a supply of tinctures to make this one. I recommend making a 100–200 millilitre supply of each of the five (licorice, marshmallow, ginger, thyme and calendula) using the instructions on page 57. Make them at a strength of 1:4, then store them in individual bottles, ready for use in remedies such as this one.

## HOW TO

**Step 1** Heat the water and glycerine in a bowl over a water bath, until the glycerine is completely dissolved, then leave to cool.

**Step 2** Pour into a sterile spray bottle, then measure out two teaspoons of each of the five tinctures and pour into the water and glycerine mixture.

**Step 3** Replace the lid. Shake well before each use.

Note: Because we have diluted this remedy with water, it won't last as long as the tinctures themselves. Keep in the fridge and use within one month, then make a fresh batch.

 **HERB NERD HACK** Spray bottles are easy enough to find, but if you don't have one, this remedy can also be used simply as a gargle.

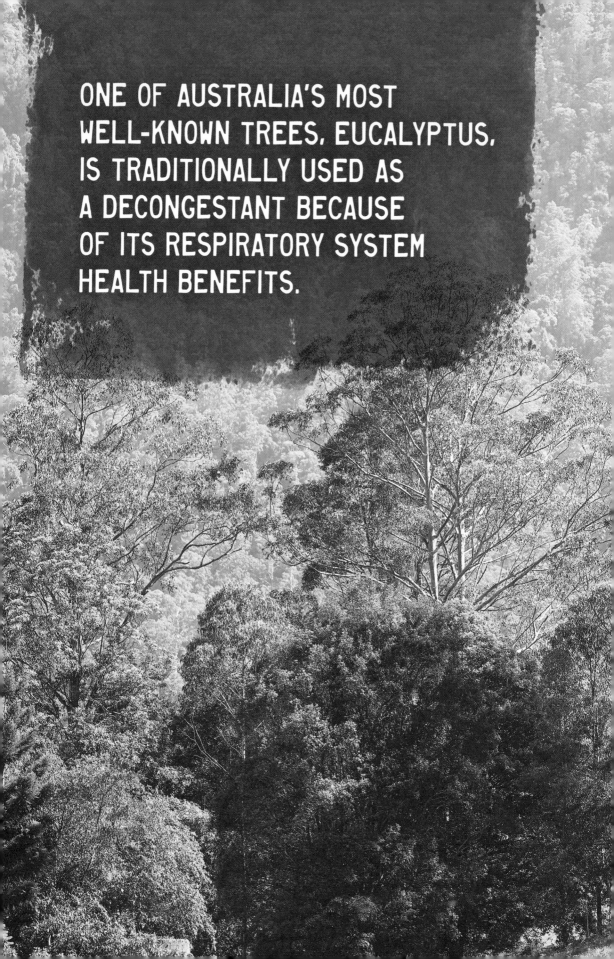

ONE OF AUSTRALIA'S MOST
WELL-KNOWN TREES, EUCALYPTUS,
IS TRADITIONALLY USED AS
A DECONGESTANT BECAUSE
OF ITS RESPIRATORY SYSTEM
HEALTH BENEFITS.

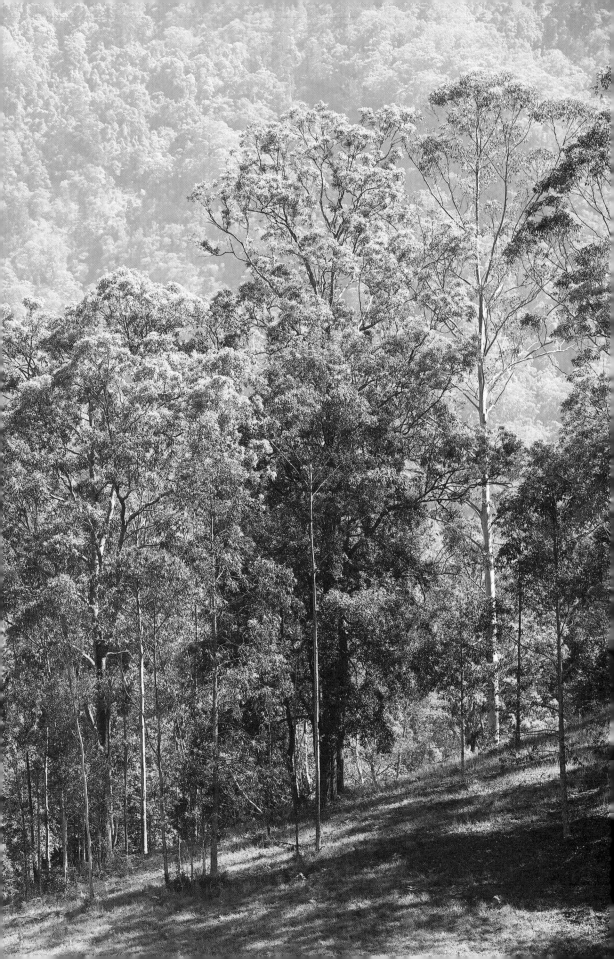

# Eucalyptus Chest Rub
## —for colds

The aroma of this liniment reminds me of being nursed back to health as a kid. Blue gum, or *Eucalyptus globulus*, is the best species because of its decongestant benefits, but any eucalyptus species will work in a pinch. If kept sealed in the fridge, this chest rub will last two or three months—just long enough to get you through winter!

## YOU WILL NEED

**For the infused eucalyptus oil**

**75 g fresh eucalyptus leaves**

**150 millilitres sweet almond oil**

**For the chest rub**

**8 g beeswax**

**100 millilitres infused eucalyptus oil (see recipe below)**

**40 drops peppermint essential oil**

**10 drops eucalyptus essential oil (optional, for added strength)**

## HOW TO

**Step 1** Grind your eucalyptus leaves in a spice grinder. Because they are fresh and still contain some water content, they will form a damp, fibrous clump rather than a powder.

**Step 2** Transfer to a large, sterile glass jar.

**Step 3** Pour over the sweet almond oil, seal and shake well to combine.

**Step 4** Place in a dark, cool place. Each day, give the jar a shake.

**Step 5** After two weeks, strain the mix through cheesecloth. Discard the solids.

**Step 6** In a double boiler, melt the beeswax (see page 72 for instructions).

**Step 7** Measure out 100 millilitres of the eucalyptus infused oil and slowly add it to the melted beeswax, stirring until well combined.

**Step 8** Remove from heat and pour into a new sterile jar.

**Step 9** Allow to cool slightly—but not to solidify—before adding your essential oils and stirring them through.

**Step 10** Rub a dollop of this on your chest whenever you've got a stagnant, chesty cold.

 **HERB NERD HACK** This recipe can be altered to make all kinds of liniments. Experiment with essential oils like cinnamon to create a remedy for muscle soreness.

# Cherry And Marshmallow Cough Syrup

*—for coughs*

Before you get too excited, I mean marshmallow root—as in from the plant *Althaea officinalis*—and not those little puffy balls of sugar. Marshmallow root soothes the throat, but it's really the wild cherry bark that shines in this recipe. We herbalists use it to reduce the cough reflex.

## YOU WILL NEED

**25 g wild cherry bark**

**25 g dried marshmallow root**

**120 millilitres food-grade vegetable glycerine**

**80 millilitres filtered water**

**200 millilitres cherry concentrate**

## HOW TO

**Step 1**  Start by grinding down your wild cherry bark and marshmallow root into smaller particles in a coffee or spice grinder.

**Step 2**  Transfer to a sterile jar, then pour in the glycerine and water. Combine well. It will probably just form one big clump in the bottle, so you might need to break it apart with a spoon, and make sure that the herbs and liquids are well combined.

**Step 3**  Seal the jar and leave in a cool, dark place for two weeks. Be sure to give the jar a shake each day.

**Step 4**  After the two weeks is up, pour in your cherry concentrate, replace the lid and shake vigorously. You want to make sure all the herb comes away from the jar and is combined with the sweet-tasting cherry liquid.

**Step 5**  Line a strainer with cheesecloth and place it over a bowl. Pour in the liquid and squeeze out all of the liquid using the back of a spoon. If you need to, put on some gloves and give the cheesecloth a real squeeze to get out all of the liquid. Discard the solids.

**Step 6**  Transfer the liquid to a sterile jar or glass bottle, seal and store in the fridge for up to a month.

**Step 7**  Measure out three teaspoons of the syrup, and take it once or twice daily.

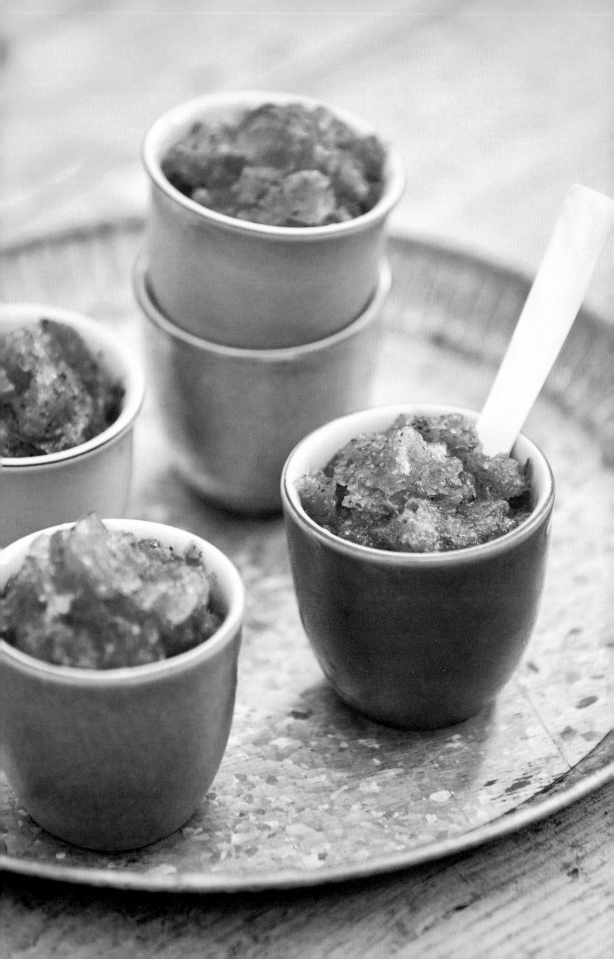

# SNIFFLE-STOP SLUSHY
## —for colds and hayfever

Whether it's seasonal allergies or the winter sniffles, there's little more annoying than a running nose. *Astringents* are herbs that act on the body's membranes and their proteins. In this instance, the effect is that they dry up the sinuses, leaving you far more comfortable, and astringents don't come much more delicious than elderflower! In this recipe I've combined it with lime because the vitamin C, along with the complementary family of compounds called bioflavonoids, acts as a natural antihistamine. *Makes four.*

## YOU WILL NEED

**9 teaspoons dried elderflower (or 8–10 fresh umbels)**

**250 millilitres (1 cup) boiling water**

**3 teaspoons honey or a few drops of stevia extract (optional)**

**2 cups watermelon, cubed and seeds removed**

**12 fresh mint leaves**

**juice from one lime**

## HOW TO

**Step 1** Using the method on page 63, make a concentrated infusion of the dried elderflower in a cup of boiling water. Stir through the honey or stevia if desired, then leave to cool.

**Step 2** Combine the watermelon, mint, lime juice and elderflower infusion in a blender, and process until smooth.

**Step 3** Freeze in an ice-cream container for 45 minutes or until half frozen. Scoop into small bowls to serve. This mixture can also be used to make popsicles. Pour into a popsicle mould and leave in the freezer until completely frozen.

**Step 4** These will keep in the freezer for one to three months before they start to become a little flavourless. My guess is they won't last that long without being devoured!

 **HERB NERD HACK** Popsicles are a fun way to get herbal medicine into fussy kids, not to mention fun-loving adults.

# REECE'S SUPERHUMAN TINCTURE

## —for cold and flu prevention

If you're looking for a go-to remedy to get you through winter, this is it. I don't understand how andrographis hasn't had its time in the spotlight like echinacea has, because, dare I say it, it's a better herb. Three teaspoons of this each day alongside a diet rich in vitamin C—think broccoli, kiwifruit, berries and citrus—will be your best bet for getting through the cold and flu season unscathed. A warning though: this is one bitter brew. As far as tinctures go, it's a definite candidate for disguising with a shot of juice.

## YOU WILL NEED

**65 g dried echinacea root**

**65 g dried andrographis**

**500 millilitres (2 cups) vodka**

## HOW TO

**Step 1** Grind the two herbs in a spice grinder and transfer to a large, sterile glass jar.

**Step 2** Pour in the vodka, replace the lid and shake well

**Step 3** Leave in a dark place for two weeks, giving the jar a shake every two to three days.

**Step 4** Strain the mixture and discard the solids.

**Step 5** Pour the liquid into a clean bottle and store in the fridge. As with other tinctures, I recommend using it within twelve months.

Note: If you prefer to make an alcohol-free version of this remedy, please use glycetract method (see page 58).

 **HERB NERD HACK** You'll know you've made a good extraction if this tincture makes your tongue tingle. That's the echinacea!

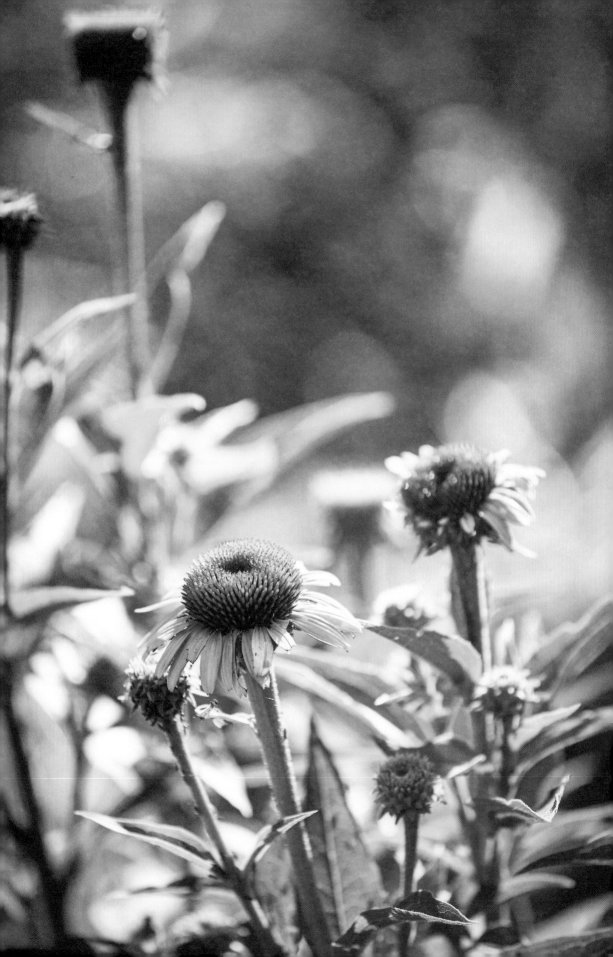

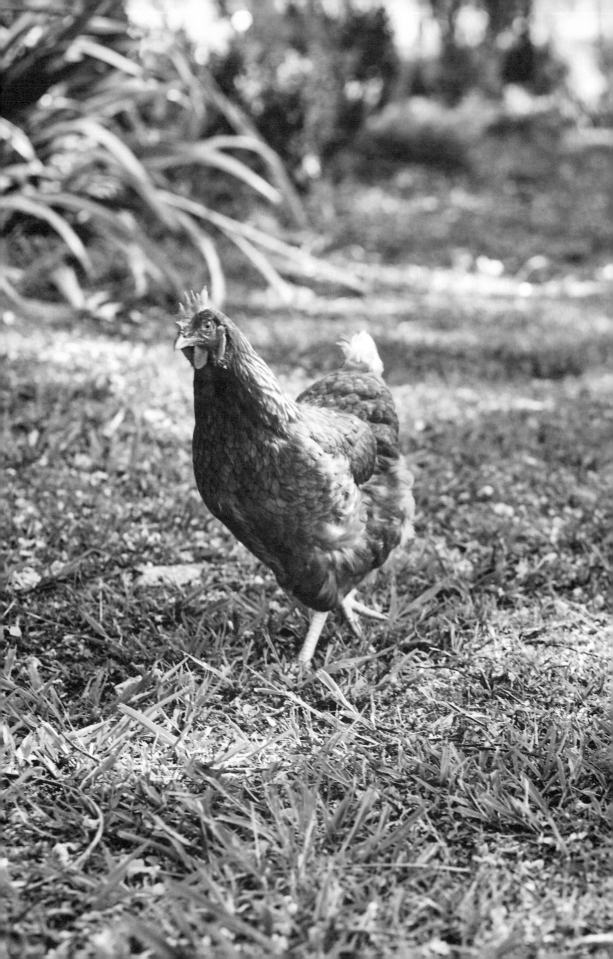

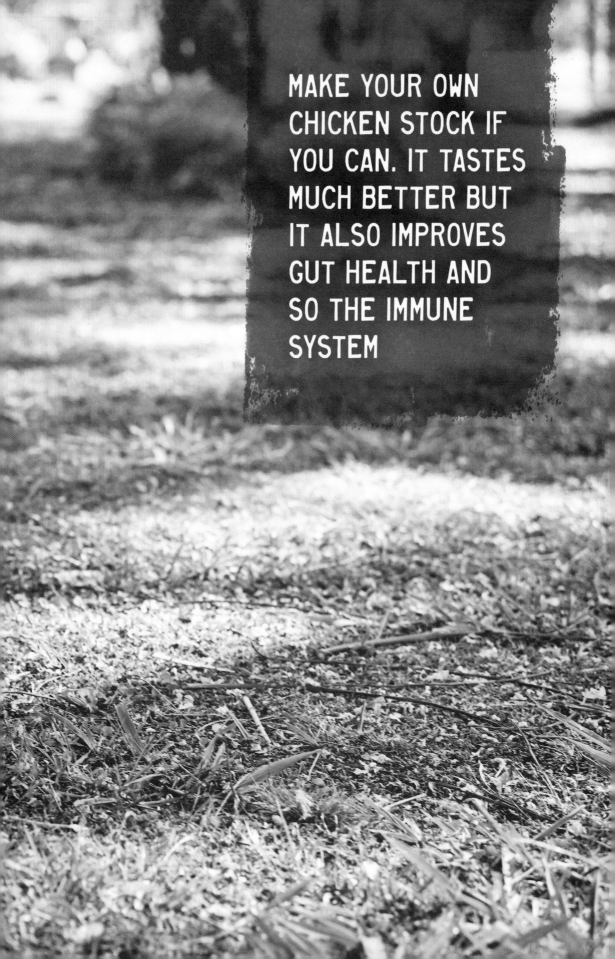

MAKE YOUR OWN
CHICKEN STOCK IF
YOU CAN. IT TASTES
MUCH BETTER BUT
IT ALSO IMPROVES
GUT HEALTH AND
SO THE IMMUNE
SYSTEM

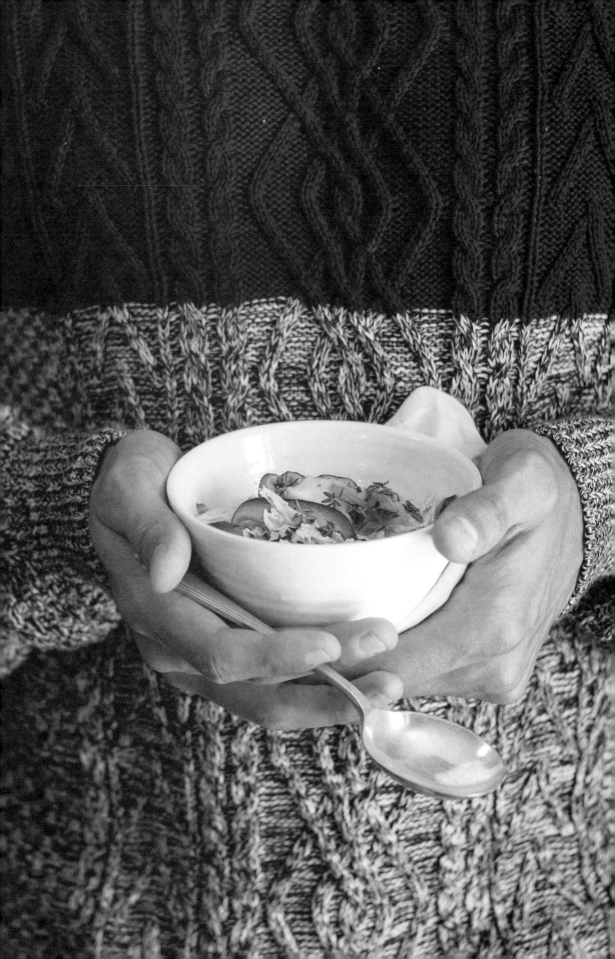

# APOTHECARY-IN-A-BOWL
## —a soup for immunity

This is my version of a comforting chicken noodle soup, with the noodles being ousted in favour of long, stringy enoki mushrooms. Mushrooms—shiitake in particular—have potent antiviral actions, and have long been used in Chinese medicine for that purpose. I've combined them with antibacterial thyme and immune-boosting garlic to deliver a soup that should be your first aid when a cold or flu hits, or just to keep your immune system well nourished through winter.

I like to make my own chicken stock for the base, as it tastes much better and improves gut health, which in turn is key to a healthy immune system. It's not an absolutely essential step, and store bought will do at a pinch, but I recommend you give it a go if you've got the time. If I make a roast chook, I always use the bones to make this broth—nothing goes to waste!

## CHICKEN STOCK

### YOU WILL NEED

**1 medium chicken carcass**

**2 carrots, peeled and roughly chopped**

**2 celery sticks, roughly chopped**

**1 brown onion, peeled and quartered**

**6 garlic cloves, peeled**

**1 bay leaf**

**½ teaspoon black peppercorns**

**3-4 thyme sprigs**

**water, to cover (approximately 3-4 litres)**

### HOW TO

**Step 1** Place all the ingredients in a large pot and bring to a boil over a high heat.

**Step 2** Reduce to a simmer, cover, then leave to cook for at least two hours. You'll need to check on it occasionally to skim off the fat from the top.

**Step 3** Once it's done, and the whole kitchen smells amazing, take the pot off the heat and remove the solids from the stock. Skim the top, then if necessary strain the stock through a sieve.

**Step 4** It's now ready to cook with, or to freeze for soups in the future!

# CHICKEN SOUP

## YOU WILL NEED

1 ½ litres (6 cups) chicken stock (see above recipe)

2 chicken breasts, skin removed

1 red onion, peeled and grated

3 teaspoons coconut oil

4 garlic cloves, crushed

1 long green chilli, seeded and finely diced

50 g shiitake mushrooms, thinly sliced

100 g enoki mushrooms, carefully separated

3 egg yolks

juice of ½ lemon

½ teaspoon ground red chilli

sea salt and black pepper, to taste

12 thyme sprigs and lemon wedges, to serve

*Makes 4 serves*

## HOW TO

**Step 1**  In a large pot, bring the stock to a boil over a high heat. Add the chicken breasts, then reduce to a simmer. Poach, covered, for 15 minutes, then remove the breasts from the stock and shred with a fork. Set the meat aside, and leave the stock gently simmering away.

**Step 2**  Meanwhile, place the grated onion in some cheesecloth and squeeze gently to remove excess moisture. If you don't have any cheesecloth, a sieve and the back of a wooden spoon will do just fine.

**Step 3**  Heat 1 teaspoon of coconut oil in a heavy-bottomed frying pan. Add the onion and cook over a medium heat for 3 minutes, then set aside.

**Step 4**  Add the other two teaspoons of coconut oil to the frying pan, then the garlic and green chilli. Cook for 30 seconds over a medium heat, then add the shiitake mushrooms. Cook for 2 minutes, stirring continuously, then add the enoki mushrooms. These won't need much time to soften, so you can take the pan off the heat and just stir well until all of the ingredients are combined.

**Step 5**  Add the onions, garlic, green chilli and mushrooms to the stock, then leave to simmer for 10 minutes. Return the chicken meat to the pot and stir the soup until all is well combined.

**Step 6**  In a small bowl, whisk together the eggs yolks and lemon juice. Add one ladle full of the stock to the bowl, being careful to avoid adding any solids, and whisk well.

**Step 7**  Slowly pour the contents of the bowl back into the soup pot. Keep whisking, and be sure the soup keeps simmering gently but doesn't come to a boil. We don't want the egg mix to curdle. Stir for a minute or two as the soup thickens, then turn off the heat.

**Step 8**  Stir in the red chilli, and season with salt and pepper.

**Step 9**  Serve each delicious bowl decorated with thyme sprigs and a lemon wedge.

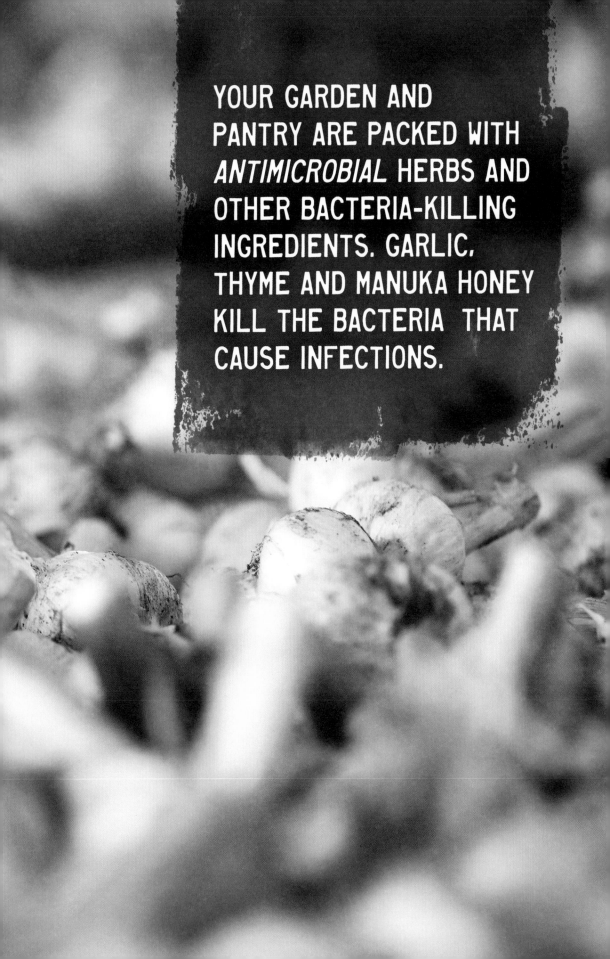

YOUR GARDEN AND PANTRY ARE PACKED WITH *ANTIMICROBIAL* HERBS AND OTHER BACTERIA-KILLING INGREDIENTS. GARLIC, THYME AND MANUKA HONEY KILL THE BACTERIA THAT CAUSE INFECTIONS.

# Horseradish Cream
## —for blocked sinuses

*Mucolytic* herbs break down mucous in the sinuses. Mucous may not be anyone's favourite topic, but uncomfortable, blocked sinuses are something we all want a cure for. Of all the mucolytics, horseradish is my favourite. It liquefies the build-up in the sinuses, so that you can breathe more easily. Use it for relief during a nasty cold, or if you suffer from nasal congestion due to allergy.

This is my mum's recipe for a yummy horseradish cream, which can be spread liberally over your meals to deliver a therapeutic dose of food as medicine.

## YOU WILL NEED

**70 g fresh horseradish, finely grated**

**200 g crème fraiche (or your favourite dairy-free substitute)**

**2 teaspoons Dijon mustard**

**squeeze of lemon juice**

**sea salt and freshly ground black pepper, to taste**

## HOW TO

**Step 1** In a small bowl, mix the grated horseradish through the crème fraiche.

**Step 2** Add the mustard and lemon juice and combine well.

**Step 3** Season with salt and pepper.

## HOW I USE IT

Horseradish cream is a classic accompaniment to steak, but not being a red meat eater myself, I prefer to enjoy it with a hearty serve of roast vegetables. Carrots, beetroot and parsnip all taste great with a spoonful of horseradish cream, and have the added benefit of delivering vitamin A to build-up your immune system.

## OR AS A DIP?

This horseradish cream can easily be turned into a delicious dip, served with crunchy veggie sticks. Make the cream according to the above recipe, and add:

**1 Lebanese cucumber, peeled, seeded and finely chopped**

**1 garlic clove, crushed**

 **HERB NERD HACK** If you're new to horseradish and its zing is a little too much for you, adding a splash of apple cider vinegar to it after grating will stop the heat from developing further.

# BUG-BUSTER GARGLE
## —for throat infections

Your garden and pantry are packed with *antimicrobial* herbs and other bacteria-killing ingredients. Garlic, thyme and manuka honey have all been shown to kill the bacteria that cause infections. You don't need anything too fancy for this one, which is good because you'll want to make a batch as soon as your throat begins to feel scratchy, then use it two or three times daily until you no longer need it.

## YOU WILL NEED

**6 thyme sprigs**

**1 small brown onion, peeled and grated**

**4 garlic cloves, crushed**

**60 millilitres (¼ cup) apple cider vinegar**

**3 teaspoons manuka honey**

## HOW TO

**Step 1**  Strip the leaves from the thyme stalks and crush them in a mortar and pestle. Transfer to a small bowl.

**Step 2**  Add the onion and garlic, then pour over the apple cider vinegar.

**Step 3**  Vigorously stir through the manuka honey, and transfer the mixture to a small jar. Seal and place in the fridge for at least four hours, or ideally overnight.

**Step 4**  Remove from the fridge, strain through cheesecloth and discard the solids. Store in an amber bottle in the fridge and use within the week.

**Step 5**  Take a swig at first sight of a throat infection and gargle for a minute or two—or for as close to it as you can manage! Do not swallow.

 Rinse out your mouth with water each time you use this one, to protect your teeth from any damage the vinegar may cause to their enamel. This also might be the time to whip out a few sprigs of parsley to chew on afterwards, to neutralise that garlic breath.

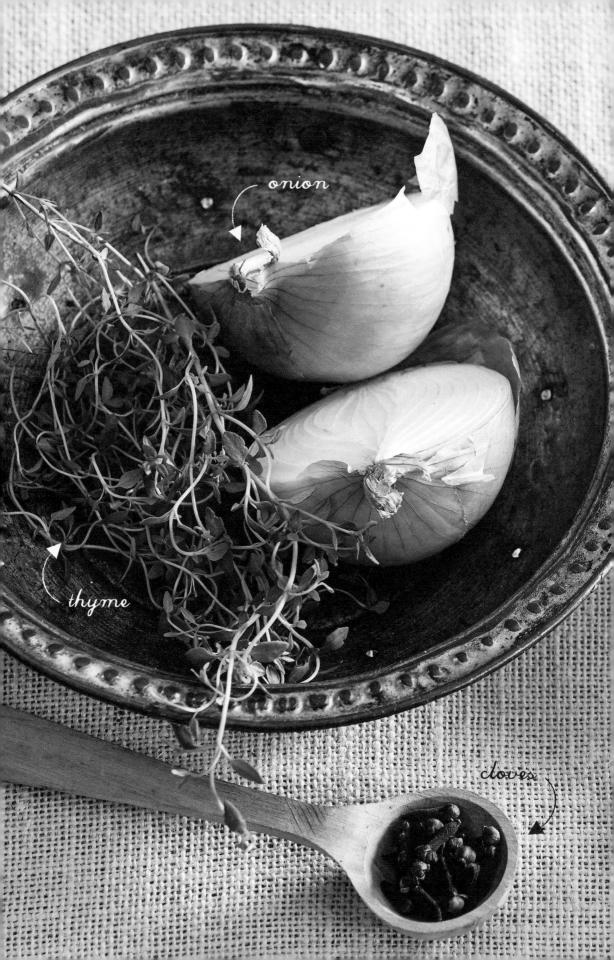

onion

thyme

cloves

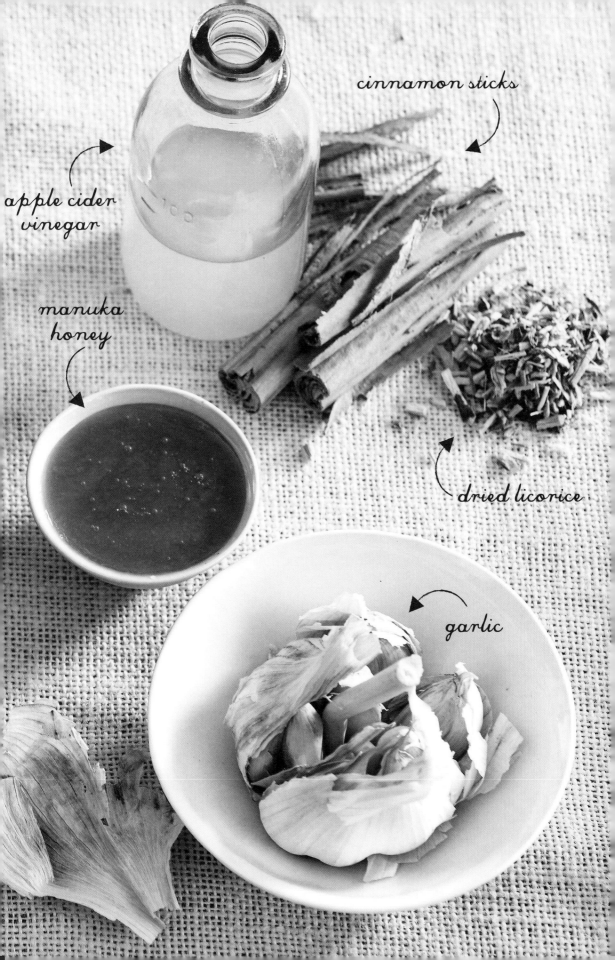

cinnamon sticks

apple cider
vinegar

manuka
honey

dried licorice

garlic

# HERBAL HOT TODDY
## —for cold and flu relief

Before you get too excited, this is my non-alcoholic version of a hot toddy. It has the same comforting taste, minus any alcohol that might lower the immune response. Licorice delivers the sweetness without any actual sugar, and soothes the throat on the way down. We've also got a healthy hit of vitamin C in the lemon juice and the cloves that act as a gentle numbing agent against any soreness.

Remember that this remedy is one to ease your symptoms, but won't do much in the way to treat the infection. My suggestion is to combine this with whichever of the *antimicrobial* and *immune-boosting* remedies you like from this chapter. *Makes one drink.*

## YOU WILL NEED

**1 teaspoon rooibos tea leaves (or one tea bag)**

**1 teaspoon dried licorice root**

**cinnamon stick, whole**

**1–2 cloves**

**juice of ½ lemon**

**500 millilitres (2 cups) water**

**slice of lemon, to serve**

## HOW TO

**Step 1** Place the rooibos tea leaves, licorice root, cinnamon stick and cloves in a small, heavy-bottomed saucepan.

**Step 2** Add the lemon juice and water, and bring the mixture to a boil over a high heat.

**Step 3** Lower the heat, and continue to simmer with the lid on for 5 minutes.

**Step 4** Strain into a big mug, and add the lemon slice. I also like to transfer the cinnamon stick across to the mug so it continues to infuse while I sip.

 **HERB NERD HACK** If you decide to add a splash of spiced rum, I won't tell anyone.

Note: Omit the licorice in this one if you have high blood pressure, and sweeten with stevia instead.

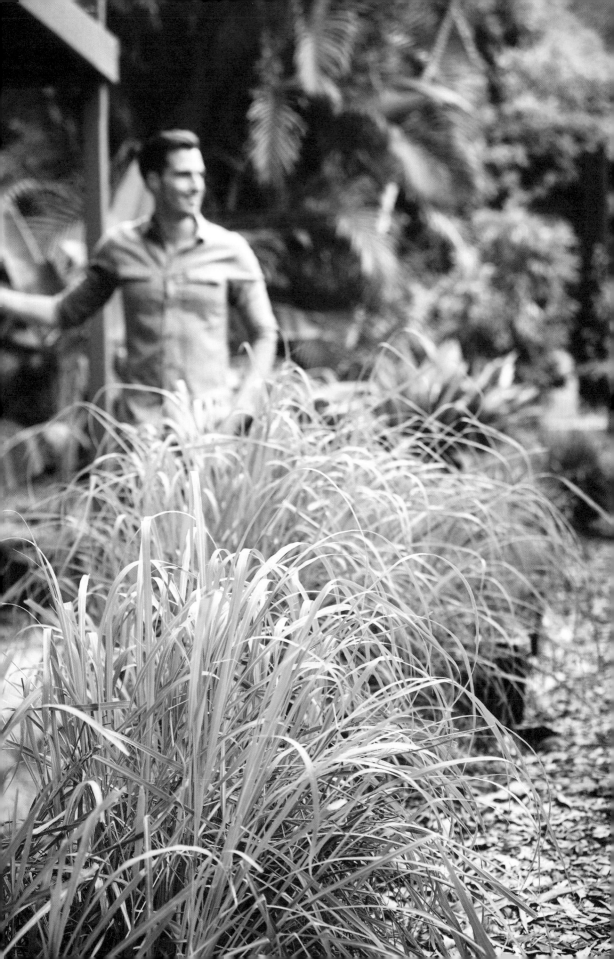

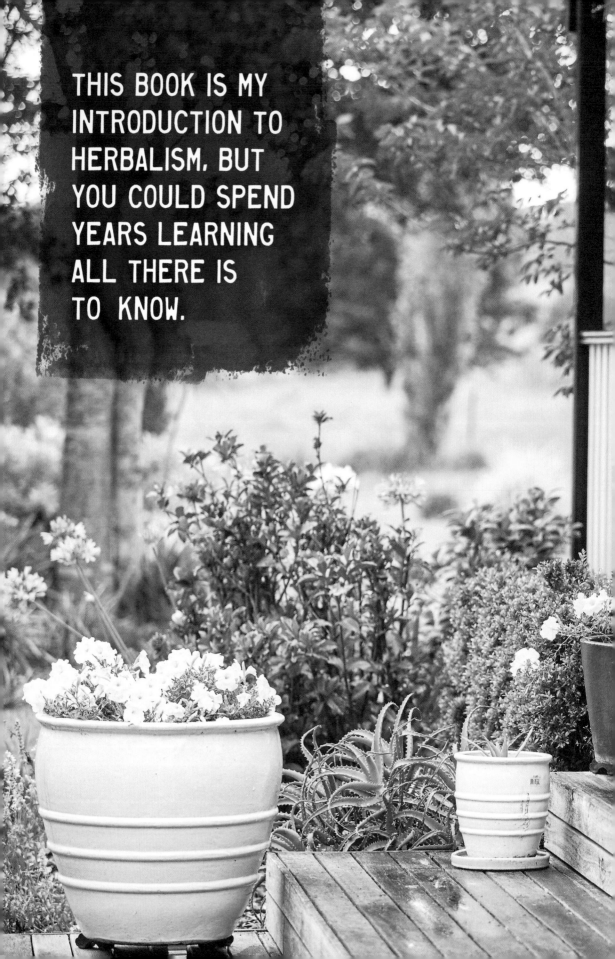

THIS BOOK IS MY
INTRODUCTION TO
HERBALISM, BUT
YOU COULD SPEND
YEARS LEARNING
ALL THERE IS
TO KNOW.

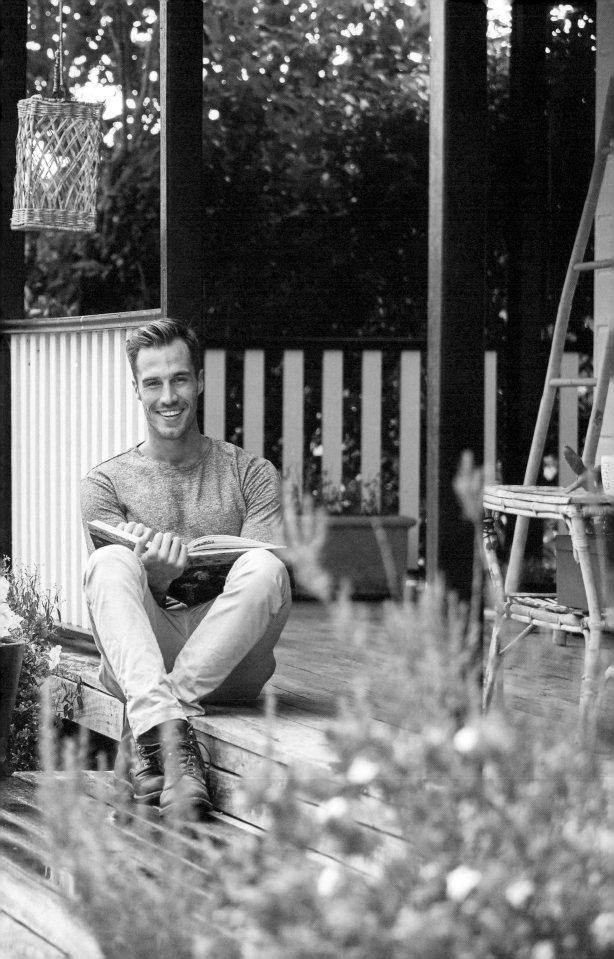

# WHAT NEXT?

**IF YOU'RE LOOKING** to discover more about the world of herbal medicine, there are plenty of resources out there to continue your research. I've listed some of my favourites below to get you started:

• *The British Herbal Pharmacopoeia* is the bible for Western herbal medicine. It covers 169 of Europe's best-known medicinal herbs, including how to identify them and their traditional uses. It can be very dry at times—it's essentially an encyclopedia—so it is probably only suited to those who want to really sink their teeth into the topic. Head to http://bhma.info to find a copy.

• *Herbal Manufacturing: How to Make Medicine from Plants* by one of my all-time favourite lecturers and wonderful naturopath Jenny Adams, and her colleague Eleanor Tan, is a self-published guide to creating all kinds of remedies. There are some specific recipes, but where this book really shines is in its thorough description of the principles and practices behind making the remedies, so that you can substitute your own favourite herbs—perhaps based on your learnings from the pharmacopoeia! You'll need to find a local natural medicine college and peruse their public bookshop for this title, as it's mostly used as a textbook. Alternatively, it can be found online at https://www.endeavourbookstore.com.au/

• If growing guides are what you're after, you can't go past Mim Beim's *Grow Your Own Medicine: A Guide to Growing Health-giving Plants in Your Own Backyard*. Mim is an Australian herbalist and used to be the Head of Naturopathy for the Australian Traditional Medicine Society (ATMS). It's a wonderful book to have on your shelves for a quick reference, and is widely available.

• If all these seem a little heavy, James Wong's *Grow Your Own Drugs* series—companions to a television series of the same name—is a wonderful, playful exploration of herbal medicine. James is an ethnobotanist, and so approaches the topic from a different angle than that of a health practitioner, giving a fresh take on it all! Like Mim Beim's titles, his books are fairly easy to come by.

• Lastly, Margo Maronne's *The Organic Pharmacy: The Complete Guide to Natural Health and Beauty* is perhaps the most readable entry-level book to natural health that I've come across. I discovered it while living in London, even before I had taken my first step towards becoming a naturopath. You'll need to order it from http://www.theorganicpharmacy.com

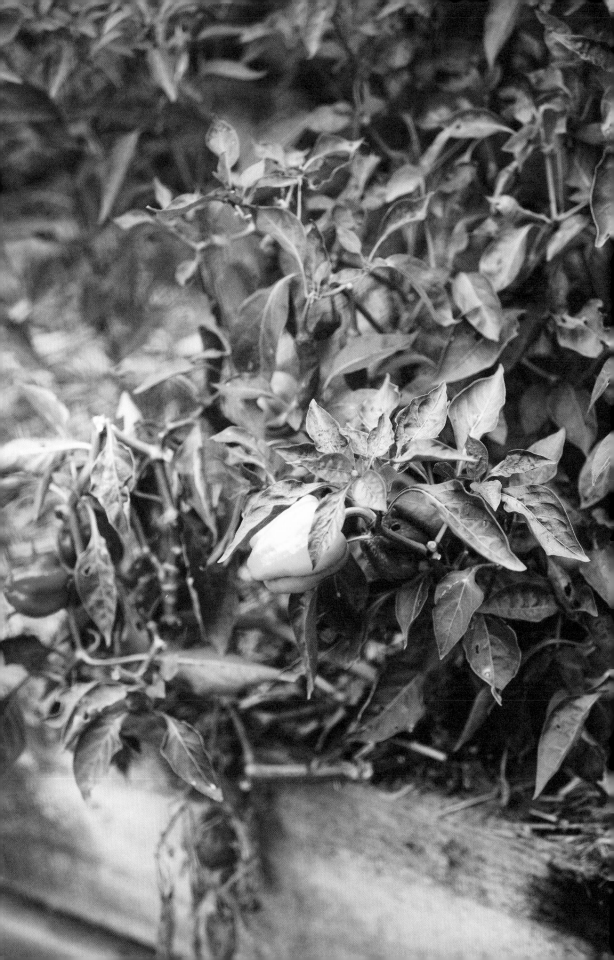

# STOCKISTS

**WHILE TURMERIC AND** garlic may be fairly easy to find at your local supermarket, there are other, more obscure herbs and ingredients that you may want to find as your apothecary grows. Even a seasoned herb nerd may find him or herself in a pinch, where they need a herb that isn't in their personal stores. In those instances, or if you're just starting out, there is always somewhere you can find a dried alternative to growing your own. Health food stores are a good place to start, but failing that the internet will usually have an answer for you. Here in Australia, some of my favourite stockists include:

Austral Herbs: www.australherbs.com.au

Southern Light Herbs: www.southernlightherbs.com.au

Melbourne Food Depot: www.melbournefooddepot.com

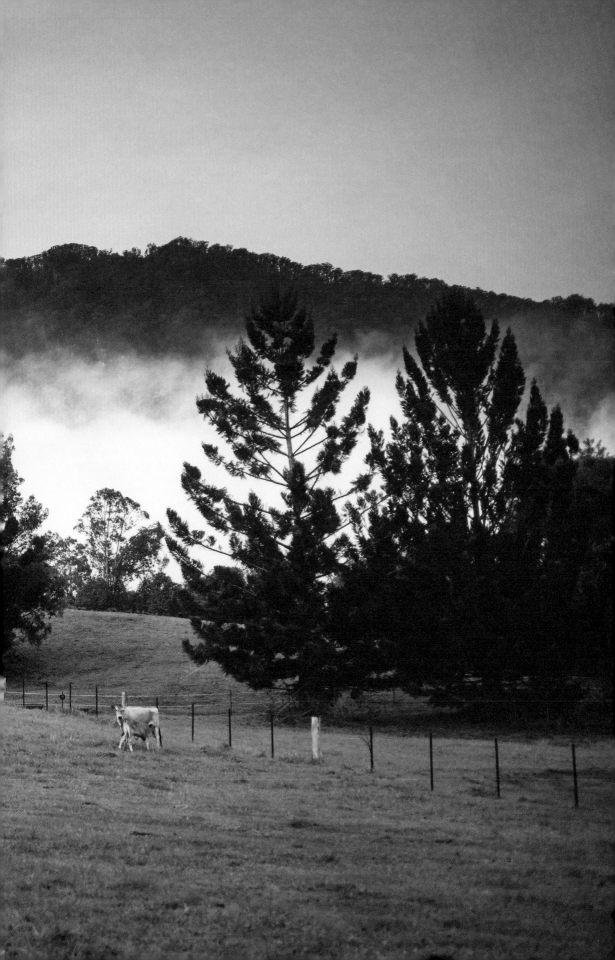

# GLOSSARY

I KNOW I'VE used a bunch of funny words in this book, so I thought I'd make it a bit easier for you by creating this little reference. After all, speaking 'herb nerd' is almost like speaking another language, so I wanted to make sure you had all the lingo down pat to talk the talk as well as you now walk the walk.

Learning how to classify plants according to their actions was my first lesson in herbalism—even before I learnt about the herbs themselves! It's a useful tool for communicating the medicinal properties of an ingredient, and will be useful as you continue to build your knowledge base and revitalise the ancient art of herbal remedies.

**Adaptogen:** A substance that increases the body's resistance to stress from both internal and external sources, and supports normal physiological function—especially in regards to hormonal regulation e.g. withania.

**Antitussive:** A herb or ingredient that decreases the severity of a cough e.g. wild cherry bark. Note that sometimes it's better to let a cough play out and not interrupt it, especially if it's a productive one.

**Anxiolytic:** An ingredient traditionally used to reduce feelings of mild anxiety e.g. lavender, passion flower.

**Aphrodisiac:** You likely know this one already. It's a food or herb consumed for its ability to increase feelings of sexual desire e.g. Korean ginseng and damiana.

**Astringent:** A substance that tightens or constricts mucous membranes such as the skin or digestive linings e.g. elderflower.

**Carminative:** A herb that reduces tightness in the muscle tissue lining the gut, so as to soothe a digestive system spasm or pain. Use these in cases of bloating and indigestion e.g. peppermint, fennel seed.

**Demulcent:** Any substance that has a soothing effect on mucous membranes like the skin, gut or respiratory tract e.g. slippery elm.

**Expectorant:** Unlike antitussives, expectorants are believed to strengthen the cough reflex so as to help you get it 'up and out' e.g. licorice.

**Glycetract:** A basic herbal extract using a mixture of food-grade vegetable glycerine and water in place of alcohol, which is used in tinctures. Glycetracts are a non-alcoholic alternative to tinctures.

**Hypnotic:** Also called soporifics, hypnotic herbs help bring on drowsiness or induce sleep e.g. hops, valerian. They're a bit of a favourite of mine.

**Mucolytic:** If you've got sinuses or a throat full of a build-up of thick, stagnant mucous, a mucolytic can be used to liquefy it e.g. horseradish. They pair nicely with expectorants.

**Nervine:** This is a beautiful term from the traditional texts that refers to a substance used to strengthen the nervous system in tone and in vigour. Such herbs are particularly useful in the 'wired but tired', the stressed and the otherwise frazzled among us e.g. oats, gotu kola.

**Thymoleptic:** Another beauty. If a herb is thymoleptic, it is used to elevate mood e.g. St John's Wort.

**Vulnerary:** This term is reserved for herbs used topically. It indicates that an ingredient may improve or support wound healing e.g. calendula.

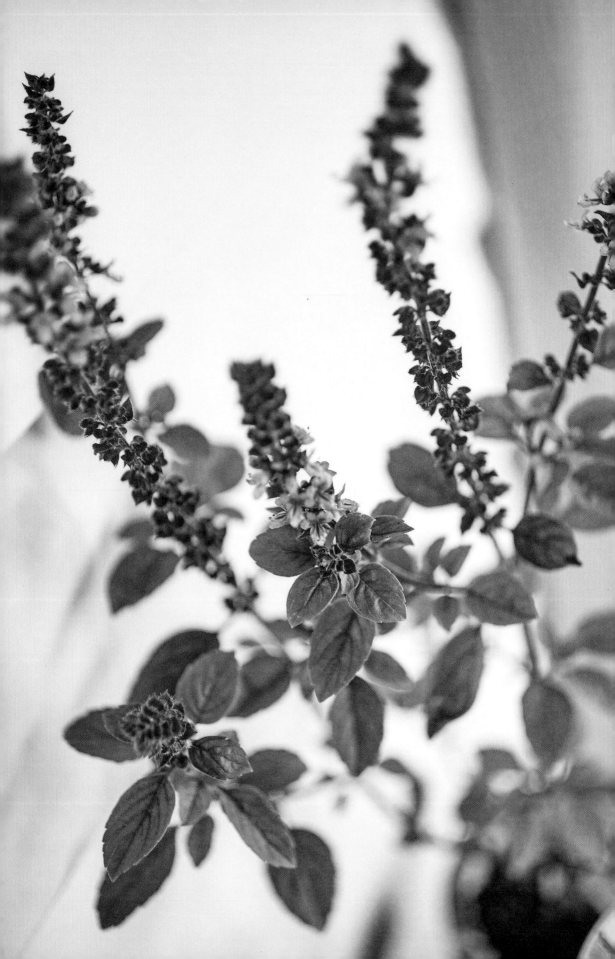

# THANK YOU

**MY NAME MIGHT** be the one printed on the cover, but in truth *The Garden Apothecary* came about because of so many more people.

Firstly, it simply wouldn't have been written if it wasn't for my monumentally supportive family and friends. Writing a book—especially a first book—takes a lot of stamina, and most of mine can be attributed to the encouragement and support of some pretty amazing people.

**Pop:** thank you for passing on your green thumb, and for all the gooseberries.

**Mr John Webb:** you let me skip class to practice my writing and storytelling skills in the library. I wouldn't have thought writing books was even an option for me without your encouragement all those years ago.

**Andree Semmens:** thank you not only for being such a knowledgeable (and often hilarious) teacher at Endeavour College of Natural Health, but also for taking the time to review my words and give your expert guidance on my manuscript.

**Lola Berry:** all of the above lessons might have amounted to nothing had you not taught me to chase my dreams relentlessly. You showed me anything is possible with a big idea and a lot of work.

**Nick Hardcastle:** Nicko, you are a legend, and one of the first people who saw potential in this herb nerd. You, Devon and Henrik were the Hollywood dream team!

**Tim, Amy and Maggie:** the kind of love and friendship you have shown me over the years still astounds me. You guys are family. Thank you for the laughs, the adventures and—unforgettably—for picking me up when I fell.

**Mum:** your belief in me seems limitless, even when my own falters. Thank you for your constant inspiration—even if you do still run rings around me in the kitchen.

In a more practical sense, this book came about because of the hard work of some phenomenally talented and passionate individuals. I'm lucky to be able to work alongside some of the best.

**Simone Landes:** I've never known anyone who works as hard as you do, Sim. In our very first meeting I said 'I want to write a book'. You didn't bat an eyelid, replied with a matter-of-fact 'OK', and we never looked back.

**Jo Mackay:** when Sim introduced us, I think it took me about twelve seconds to decide 'yes, this is the woman I want to look after my book!' You understood my vision immediately, and your passion for the project made me feel certain that my words were in safe hands. I owe a massive thanks to you, as well as to Adam, Sue, Annabel and the rest of the team at Harlequin who made this happen.

**Stuart Scott:** that has to have been one of the easiest and most fun photo shoots ever! Thanks for capturing the essence of the book so perfectly up on Moo River Farm, and to your family for their wonderful Bellingen hospitality.

**Sarah De Nardi:** your car was nearly overflowing with props, plants and personality when you arrived on the shoot. It was a totally legendary effort that yielded beautiful results.

**Autonomy Clothing:** my favourite Aussie label! Thanks so much to Simone for supplying most of the looks in this book. You are a champion.

**Liz and Greg from Merricks Creek Organics:** your farm is absolutely incredible and I can't think of anywhere better to have shot *The Garden Apothecary*—and a special mention to Jill the Kelpie for her enthusiastic participation!

**Suzie at Cottonwood Cottage:** the very first photo (and one of my favourites) was taken on your property, and it couldn't have been a more perfect start to the shoot. I'll definitely be back next time I'm in Bello!

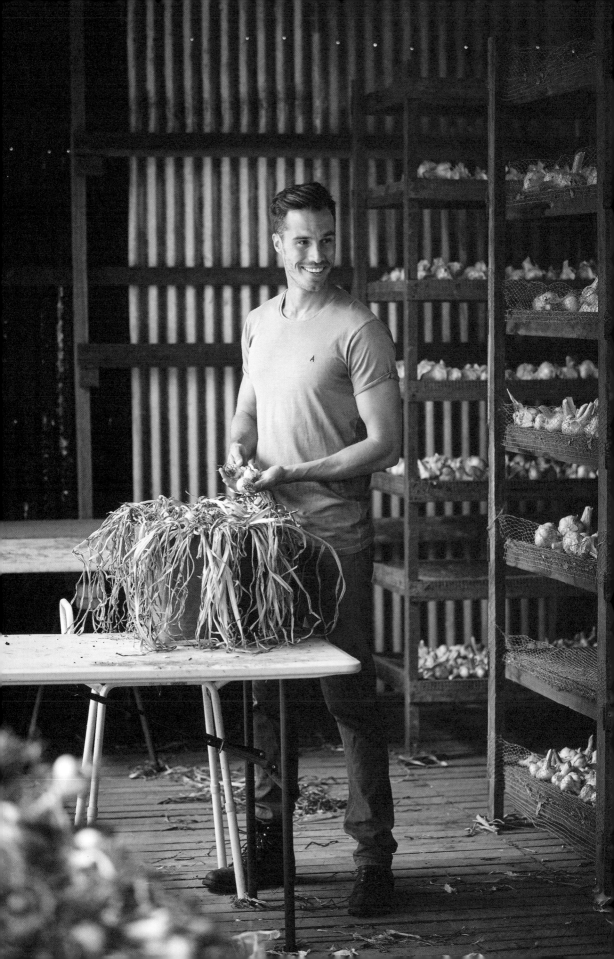

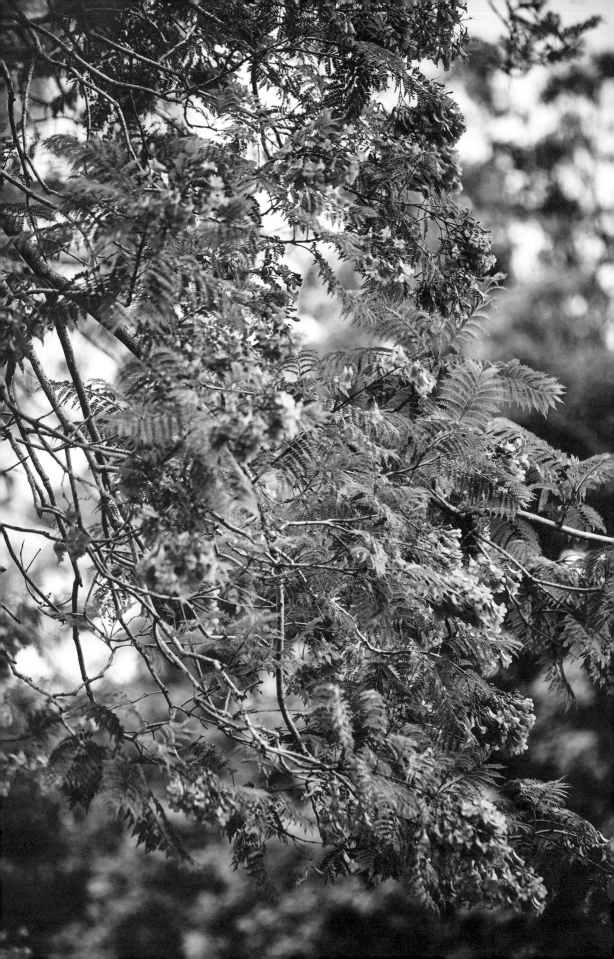

# INDEX

References to content in the glossary are indexed with a 'g' following the page number.

6 pm blend 121

acne *see* skin health
adaptogens 176g
allergies 42, 66 *see also* respiratory health
aloe vera 34–35
    Aloe eye gel 72
    Aloe ice 84
    Gut-healing smoothie 136
andrographis
    Reece's superhuman tincture 156
Anti-inflammitea 132
antitussives 176g
anxiety 40, 112–113 *see also* sleep; stress
    Meditation candle 115
    Sleep potion 126
    valerian root and 51
anxiolytics 176g
aphrodisiacs 92–93, 176g
    Libido-boost shot 97
Apothecary-in-a-bowl 161–162
appetite 47
arthritis 51
ashwaganda
    Sleep potion 126
astringents 176g
avocados
    Choc-avo face mask 80

basil
    'Forget-me-not' salsa verde 104
Bedtime chai 114
beeswax 24
Belly jellies 143–144
berries *see* strawberries
bloating *see* digestive health
books 172
bowel health *see* digestive health
brahmi 35
Bug-buster gargle 165
buying herbs 20, 23, 47–51, 174

cacao powder
    Choc-avo face mask 80
    Choc-coffee skin scrub 81
    Maca-macadamia chocolate bark 103
    Overnight oats 94
calendula 35, 38, 42
    Aloe ice 84
    Organo-oil 74
    Skin repair body cream 68
    Sore throat spray 149
candles 113, 115
cardamon
    Anti-inflammitea 132
    Bedtime chai 114

carminatives 177g
cayenne pepper
    Matcha warrior 96
chamomile (essential oil)
    Meditation candle 115
chamomile (flowers) 38–39, 42
    Aloe ice 84
    Cleopatra's bath mylk 87
    Lemon balm iced tea 125
    Skin repair body cream 68
cheesecloth 24
cherry bark
    Cherry and marshmallow cough syrup 153
chicken
    Chicken soup 162
    Chicken stock 161
'Chill pill' bath bomb 118
chillies 38
    Chicken soup 162
    Maca-macadamia chocolate bark 103
Choc-avo face mask 80
cholesterol reduction 48–50
    Overnight oats 94
cinnamon
    Anti-inflammitea 132
    Bedtime chai 114
    Eucalyptus chest rub 152
    Herbal hot toddy 168
Cleopatra's bath mylk 87
cloves
    Herbal hot toddy 168
    Herbal mouthwash 89
coconut oil *see* infused oils
coconuts
    Cleopatra's bath mylk 87
    Overnight oats 94
coffee
    Choc-coffee skin scrub 81
colds *see* respiratory health
constipation *see* digestive health
containers 24
coriander seeds
    Digestive dukkah 142
coughs *see* respiratory health
cramps 48–49
creams 19, 23–24
    Skin repair body cream 68
cumin seeds
    Digestive dukkah 142

daisy family 42 *see also* calendula; chamomile; dandelion; echinacea; feverfew
damiana
    Libido-boost shot 97
dandelion 42, 47–48
decoctions 19–20, 48, 63
    A digestive decoction 133
    Anti-inflammitea 132
    Herbal hot toddy 168
    Nourish and nurture 121

decongestants *see* respiratory health
demulcents 177g
A digestive decoction 133
Digestive dukkah 142
digestive health 47–49, 130–144
    peppermint and 41
    turmeric and 51
DIY herb drying 45
DIY planter boxes 31–32
drinks *see also* tea
    Gut-healing smoothie 136
    Hibiscus and raspberry kefir 137
    Libido-boost shot 97
drying herbs 45

echinacea 42
    Reece's superhuman tincture 156
eczema *see* skin health
elderflower 48
    Sniffle-stop slushy 155
emotions *see* mood
emulsifying wax 23–24
energy *see* fatigue
equipment 24
Eucalyptus chest rub 152
expectorants 177g

face masks
    Choc-avo face mask 80
    Honey-oat face mask 77
    Kiwi-berry face mask 76
fatigue 92–93
    green tea and 50
    Maca-macadamia chocolate bark 103
    Matcha warrior 96
    Mum's best mate 120
    Nourish and nurture 121
    'Pep me up' peppermint mist 101
fennel seeds 48
    A digestive decoction 133
    Digestive dukkah 142
feverfew 42
    Fresh feverfew tea 107
flatulence *see* digestive health
fluid extracts *see* tinctures
food 35, 38–39, 47–49, 51 *see also* drinks
    Apothecary-in-a-bowl 161–162
    Belly jellies 143–144
    Digestive dukkah 142
    Hangover sherbet 100
    Horseradish cream 164
    Maca-macadamia chocolate bark 103
    Overnight oats 94
    Sniffle-stop slushy 155
'Forget-me-not' salsa verde 104
Fresh feverfew tea 107

gardening *see* growing herbs
garlic 48–49
    Bug-buster gargle 165

German chamomile *see* chamomile
ginger 49
    Anti-inflammitea 132
    Ginger pastilles 138
    Hangover sherbet 100
    Sore throat spray 149
ginseng
    Libido-boost shot 97
glassware
    choosing and sterilising 24
glossary 176–177
glycerine 19, 23, 50, 58, 177g
gotu kola
    'Forget-me-not' salsa verde 104
green tea 49–50
    Green tea toner 83
    Herbal mouthwash 89
    Matcha warrior 96
grinding spices 24
growing herbs 20, 28–42
Gut-healing smoothie 136

hair health 66, 88
hangovers 49
    Hangover sherbet 100
hayfever *see* respiratory health
headaches
    Fresh feverfew tea 107
Herbal hot toddy 168
Herbal mouthwash 89
herbs
    buying 20, 23, 47–51, 174
    drying 45
    growing 28–42
    reasons for using 11–14
hibiscus
    Hibiscus and orange blossom jellies 143–144
    Hibiscus and raspberry kefir 137
honey
    Anti-inflammitea 132
    Bug-buster gargle 165
    Honey-oat face mask 77
hops
    Sleep potion 126
horseradish 39
    Horseradish cream 164
hypnotics 177g

immunity 41, 48–49
    Apothecary-in-a-bowl 161–162
    Reece's superhuman tincture 156
indigestion *see* digestive health
inflammation 49, 51
infused oils 19, 23, 38, 60
    brahmi in 35
    Eucalyptus chest rub 152
    Organo-oil 74
infusions 19–20, 38–41, 48–50, 63
    6 pm blend 121
    Fresh feverfew tea 107

Lemon balm iced tea  125
Mum's best mate  120
insomnia  *see* sleep
intestinal health  *see* digestive health

jasmine essential oil
Cleopatra's bath mylk  87
Skin repair body cream  68
joint pain  51
Anti-inflammitea  132
Joy-in-a-jar tincture  108

kefir
Hibiscus and raspberry kefir  137
kiwifruit
Gut-healing smoothie  136
Kiwi-berry face mask  76

lavender (essential oil)
'Chill pill' bath bomb  118
Green tea toner  83
Meditation candle  115
Skin repair body cream  68
lavender (flowers)  40
'Chill pill' bath bomb  118
Joy-in-a-jar tincture  108
Lemon balm iced tea  125
Nourish and nurture  121
leaky gut  *see* digestive health
lemon balm  40–41
Joy-in-a-jar tincture  108
Lemon balm iced tea  125
Lemon balm ointment  73
libido  92–93, 176g
Libido-boost shot  97
licorice root  50
A digestive decoction  133
Herbal hot toddy  168
Herbal mouthwash  89
Nourish and nurture  121
Sore throat spray  149
limes
Overnight oats  94
lip balms
Peppermint lip balm  85
liver health  47
lotions  19
Luscious locks hair mask  88

macadamia nuts
Maca-macadamia chocolate bark  103
Maca-macadamia chocolate bark  103
marshmallow
Cherry and marshmallow cough syrup  153
Sore throat spray  149
Matcha warrior  96
medication  12–13
Meditation candle  113, 115
Melissa  *see* lemon balm

memory  35
'Forget-me-not' salsa verde  104
menstruums  18–20, 23, 55
mental clarity
'Pep me up' peppermint mist  101
metabolism  38
Matcha warrior  96
migraines  *see* headaches
mint  *see also* peppermint ...
Lemon balm iced tea  125
Sniffle-stop slushy  155
mood  40, 92–93
Joy-in-a-jar tincture  108
Maca-macadamia chocolate bark  103
motherwort
Mum's best mate  120
motion sickness  *see* nausea
mouthwash
Herbal mouthwash  89
mucolytics  177g
Mum's best mate  120
muslin  24

Nature's antacid pills  139
nausea  49
Ginger pastilles  138
nervines  177g
Nourish and nurture  121
nutmeg
Bedtime chai  114
nuts  *see* macadamia nuts; pistachio nuts

oats  50
Cleopatra's bath mylk  87
Honey-oat face mask  77
Overnight oats  94
oils
essential  *see names of essential oils*
infused  *see* infused oils
ointments  19, 24
Lemon balm ointment  73
oral hygiene  89
orange blossom water
Hibiscus and orange blossom jellies  143
Organo-oil  74
Overnight oats  94

papaya
Gut-healing smoothie  136
parsley
'Forget-me-not' salsa verde  104
passionflower
Mum's best mate  120
Sleep potion  126
'Pep me up' peppermint mist  101
pepper
Anti-inflammitea  132
Chicken stock  161
peppermint (essential oil)  107

Eucalyptus chest rub 152
Luscious locks hair mask 88
'Pep me up' peppermint mist 101
Peppermint lip balm 85
peppermint (leaves) 41
A digestive decoction 133
Gut-healing smoothie 136
Herbal mouthwash 89
Peppermint belly jellies 144
period pain 49
pharmaceuticals 12–13
pineapples
Gut-healing smoothie 136
pistachio nuts
Overnight oats 94
planter boxes 31–32
pomegranate
Overnight oats 94
pots see planter boxes
preservation of remedies 55

raw cacao powder see cacao powder
Reece's superhuman tincture 156
resources 172
respiratory health 42, 48–50, 148–168
Bug-buster gargle 165
chamomile and 39
Sore throat spray 149
rooibos tea
Bedtime chai 114
Herbal hot toddy 168
rose hips
Organo-oil 74
rose petals
Mum's best mate 120
'Pep me up' peppermint mist 101
rosella see hibiscus
rosemary essential oil
Luscious locks hair mask 88
rosewater
Overnight oats 94

science 12
sinus health see respiratory health
skin health 34–35, 38–39, 49–50, 66–87
allergies 42
Skin repair body cream 68
sleep 112–113 see also anxiety; stress
Bedtime chai 114
chamomile and 38–39
lemon balm and 40–41
Sleep potion 126
valerian root and 51
slippery elm
Gut-healing smoothie 136
Nature's antacid pills 139
Sniffle-stop slushy 155
soporifics 177g
sore throats see respiratory health

spice grinders 24
St John's Wort
Joy-in-a-jar tincture 108
sterilisation of containers 24
stockists see buying herbs
strawberries
Kiwi-berry face mask 76
stress 40, 112–113 see also anxiety; sleep
6 pm blend 121
'Chill pill' bath bomb 118
Lemon balm iced tea 125
licorice root and 50
Overnight oats 94
sunburn see skin health
sweet almond oil see infused oils

tea 19–20, 49–51, 72 see also decoctions; green tea;
infusions; rooibos tea
Anti-inflammitea 132
tea tree oil
Lemon balm ointment 73
throat infections see respiratory health
thyme 41–42
Bug-buster gargle 165
Chicken soup 162
Chicken stock 161
Sore throat spray 149
thymoleptics 177g
tinctures 19, 23
brahmi in 35
Ginger pastilles 138
Herbal mouthwash 89
horseradish 39
Joy-in-a-jar tincture 108
lemon balm, valerian and hops 41
licorice root 50
making 54–58
Reece's superhuman tincture 156
Sleep potion 126
Sore throat spray 149
tiredness see fatigue
turmeric 51, 139
Anti-inflammitea 132
Digestive dukkah 142

valerian root 51
Bedtime chai 114
vegetable glycerine see glycerine
vodka see tinctures
vulneraries 177g

wax 23–24
weight loss 38, 50
witch hazel
Aloe eye gel 72
Green tea toner 83

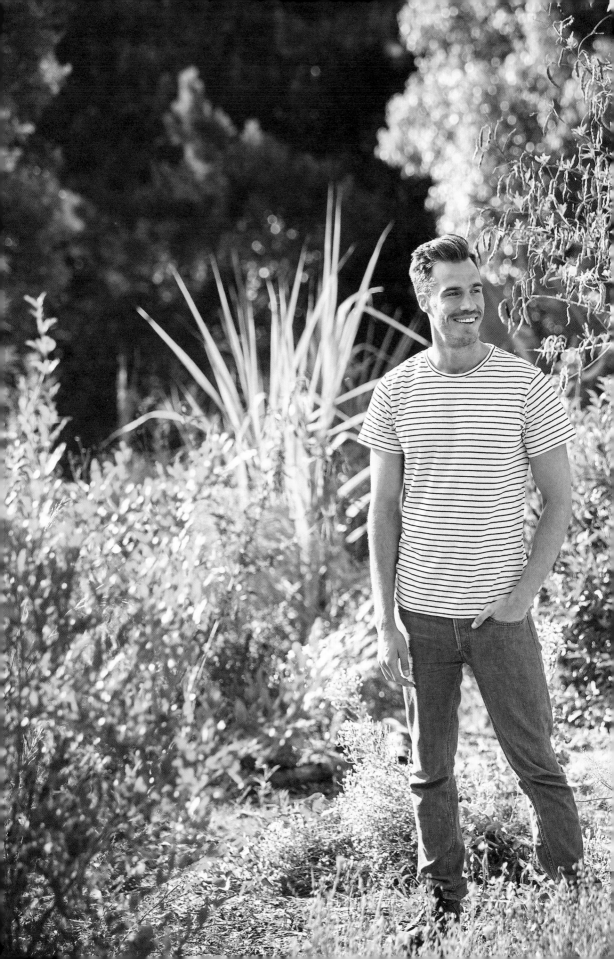

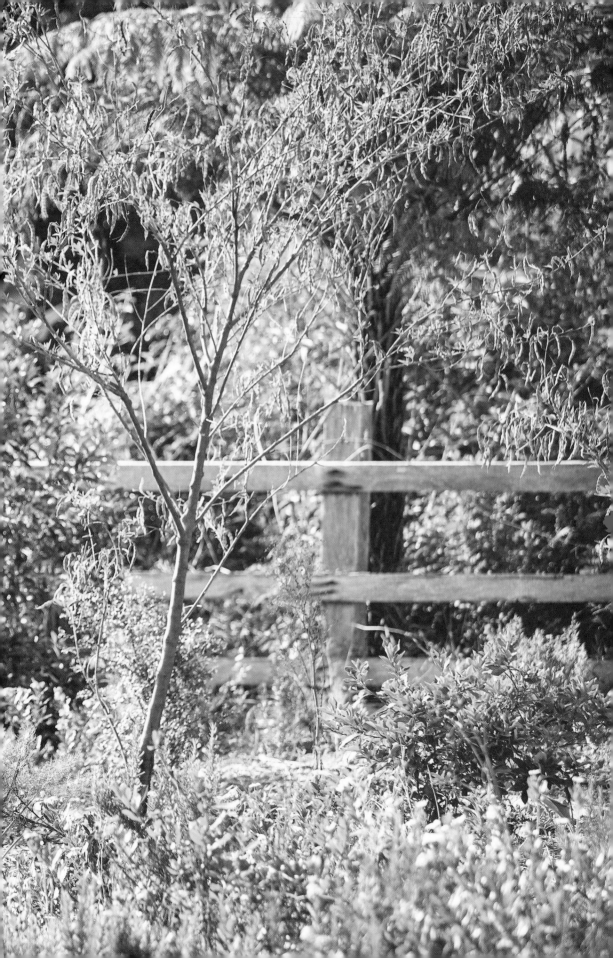

First published July 2017 by HQ Non Fiction
An imprint of Harlequin Enterprises (Australia) Pty Ltd.
Level 13, 201 Elizabeth St
SYDNEY NSW 2000
AUSTRALIA

ISBN 9781489216007

The Garden Apothecary
© Reece Carter 2017

Cover and internal design by Alicia Freile, Tango Media
Cover image and photography by Stuart Scott
except pages 69, 105 and 160 by Darren Holt
Styling by Sarah De Nardi
Printed and bound in China

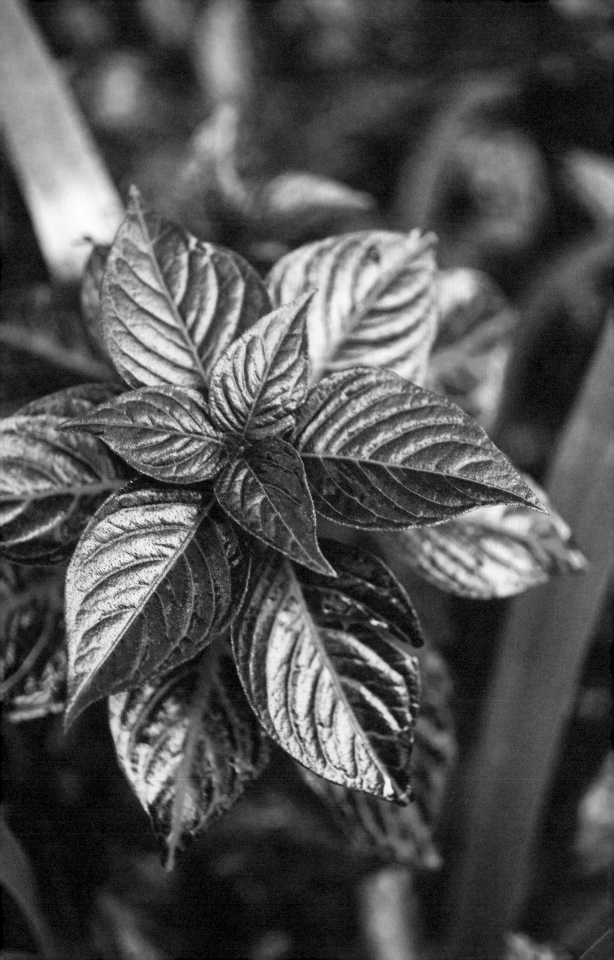

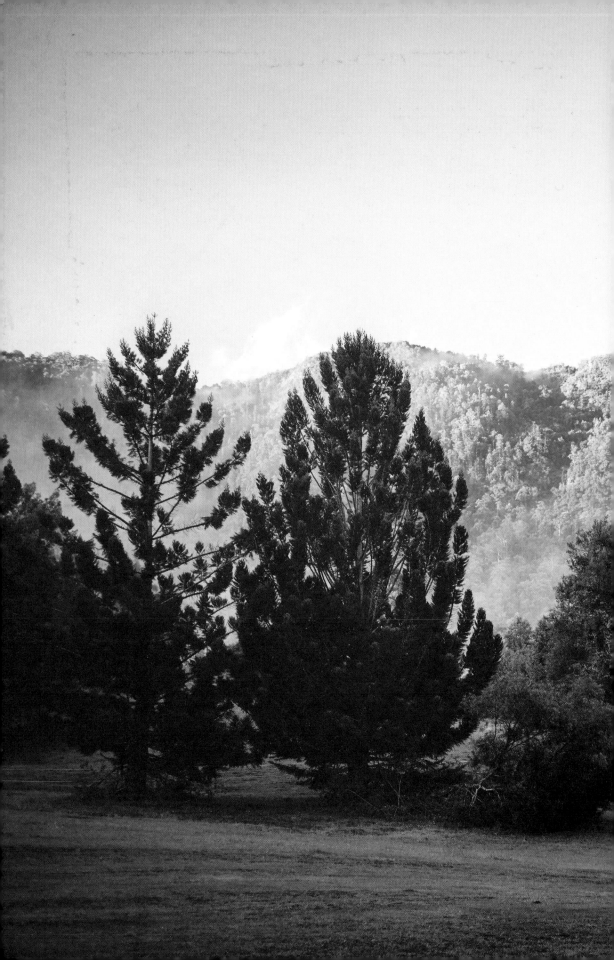